Engaging and a must-read for all wo[...]
candid, real, and inspiring. Jennifer's [...]
journey helps readers discover their *why* through personal
reflection and action steps.

SHARON McQUEEN, pastor, Family Life Church

Your Good Body is one word: extraordinary. Jennifer has
charged herself with bringing awareness to our unconscious
destructive thoughts and breathing life into loving the
journey we're on. This book challenges your thoughts and
the relationship you have with yourself. When you start
reading, Jennifer is just an author, but when you finish,
she's a friend you want to invite to your house for tea.
Absolutely *love* this book.

CHARMAINE COUSINS, PhD

After recent weight loss, this book helped me release the
mental and emotional weight that I didn't even know I
was carrying. I now know that I have a *good body*!

PAIGE LOEHR, author of *The Roots in a Woman*

Jennifer is the voice that every woman—whether 16, 46,
or 60—needs in her head! Stop letting the scale boss you or
shame you. Let this book be your new soundtrack instead.
Take it from a middle-aged mom who is exhausted by the
numbers that judge her every morning. This body is ready to
remember why it is good, beloved, and beautiful just as it is.

LISA-JO BAKER, bestselling author of *Never Unfriended* and cohost of the
podcast *Out of the Ordinary Books*

Jennifer is a powerhouse in the lane of helping women view their bodies as good. Her story and the way she models a healthy perspective has been so transformative for me, and I know it will be in the lives of her readers. I can't wait to see the freedom that breaks out in women as they come to realize God designed their bodies as good!

REBECCA GEORGE, author and host of the podcast *Radical Radiance*™

I was highly impressed, emotionally moved, inspired, and empowered after I read *Your Good Body* by Jennifer Taylor Wagner. As an emphatic goal setter and goal getter, I thoroughly enjoyed Jennifer's transparency and vulnerability as she precisely shared her weight loss journey and struggle with perfectionism and how she overcame insecurity to obtain true and sincere happiness. Not only did Jennifer open her heart and life within these pages, but I also enjoyed the exercises that are included at the end of every chapter. It made me really give thought to why I do what I do. Overall, this unique book is a must-read if you're looking for empowering inspiration, practical information, and emotional support while on a weight loss journey. I promise you it will change your life because it changed mine.

WANDA MARTIN, author of *Go for the Goal*, founder and CEO of GO FOR THE GOAL ACADEMY, and board member and goal-setting advisor of Coaches Against Childhood Obesity

Jennifer speaks right to the journey many women have walked at some time in their life. Her words inspire acceptance and love for your body as is and propel you toward being your best self in mind and body. *Your Good Body* isn't just good, it's great.

ASHLEY SOLBERG

It feels like Jennifer may have written *Your Good Body* just for me. It is personal and uplifting and has helped heal years of hurt and striving for the perfect body. This book showcases that contentment is not a number on a scale but a confidence in the body that God created specifically for you. This is a must-read for women of any age and at any point in their health journey.

MATTIE GIVENS, mattiegivens.com

"Woo-hoo!" was my first reaction as I read Jennifer Taylor Wagner's *Your Good Body: Embracing a Body-Positive Mindset in a Perfection-Focused World*. It offers readers a journey of discovery: self-compassion, grit, motivation, and insight about what holds us back from reaching for our dreams and goals and how to get unstuck and move forward. It is also packed with practical tools and tips. This is *not* the typical book on weight loss. Jennifer communicates with authenticity, empathy, and hope that draws people who have struggled with similar body image issues.

WANDA SANCHEZ, executive producer, Salem Radio Network, San Francisco; author of the multiple award-winning *Love Letters from the Edge: Meditations for Those Struggling with Brokenness, Trauma, and the Pain of Life;* monthly contributor to *The Mighty*

We are so quick to marvel in the beauty that God has created in the world around us, but we are so quick to dismiss the beauty that is our own body. Jennifer speaks the incredible truth of the incredible beauty of each individual body—that God made no mistake in the way each of us were created and that we should love and appreciate every aspect of it. This book is one that I hope females of all ages not only read once but again and again and soak in every powerful message that Jennifer so eloquently shares!

JENN RICHARDSON, CEO, Fit Couture Collection

YOUR GOOD BODY

YOUR GOOD BODY

Embracing a Body-Positive Mindset

in a Perfection-Focused World

JENNIFER TAYLOR WAGNER

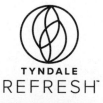

TYNDALE
REFRESH™

Think Well. Live Well. Be Well.

Visit Tyndale online at tyndale.com.

Tyndale and Tyndale's quill logo are registered trademarks of Tyndale House Ministries. *Tyndale Refresh* and the Tyndale Refresh logo are trademarks of Tyndale House Ministries. Tyndale Refresh is a nonfiction imprint of Tyndale House Publishers, Carol Stream, Illinois.

Your Good Body: Embracing a Body-Positive Mindset in a Perfection-Focused World

Cover and interior designed by Libby Dykstra

Author photo taken by Alisa Sue Photography, copyright © 2020. All rights reserved.

Edited by Karin Stock Buursma

Unless otherwise indicated, all Scripture quotations are taken from the *Holy Bible*, New Living Translation, copyright © 1996, 2004, 2015 by Tyndale House Foundation. Used by permission of Tyndale House Publishers, Carol Stream, Illinois 60188. All rights reserved.

Scripture quotations marked NIV are taken from the Holy Bible, *New International Version,*® *NIV.*® Copyright © 1973, 1978, 1984, 2011 by Biblica, Inc.® Used by permission. All rights reserved worldwide.

For information about special discounts for bulk purchases, please contact Tyndale House Publishers at csresponse@tyndale.com, or call 1-855-277-9400.

Library of Congress Cataloging-in-Publication Data

A catalog record for this book is available from the Library of Congress.

ISBN 978-1-4964-5417-1

Printed in the United States of America

27	26	25	24	23	22	21
7	6	5	4	3	2	1

To my favorite human on the planet.

For drying my eyes a hundred times as I stepped off the scale.

For ordering pizza with me late at night.

For buying me the two-piece.

For loving my love handles.

You're one-of-a-kind amazing, Phil Wagner.

I love you so very much.

TABLE OF CONTENTS

INTRODUCTION

I want to ask you a question—

How much do you weigh?

Yeesh, right? I felt you cringe. Other than perhaps, "How would you like to die?" (or something of the like), this might be the worst question anyone can ask a woman. But before you abandon this book, I promise there is a purpose to this question. In fact, why don't you save your answer, and I'll tell you mine.

Hi! I'm Jennifer. And my weight was 336.

Yes, you read that correctly. No typo here. 336 pounds. That number will forever be etched in my brain because I think about it every single day of my life. I spent years in a body that was bigger than my capacity to navigate it through a cruel world that overwhelmingly values the external over the internal. I was bullied relentlessly all through my younger years, and things got so bad that by the time I finished high school, I fled to another state to start a new life on my own. A few years later I began a massive weight-loss pursuit.

I wasn't one of those beautifully vibrant and full-of-life curvy girls who seems completely comfortable in her body. (Those weren't as common—or at least as public—back in the 1990s.) Quite the opposite. My self-esteem was a whopping *zero*, and for nineteen years of my life, I just knew there was something terribly wrong with me because of my weight. I was sure that if I *ever* cracked the code to losing weight, my life would be wonderful. Then—and only then—I would feel great, and all would be right in the world.

> I was sure that if I ever cracked the code to losing weight, my life would be wonderful. Then—and only then—I would feel great, and all would be right in the world.

Through persistence and a shift in my relationship with food and exercise, I did what most people with weight struggles want to do: I lost the weight. One hundred sixty pounds, to be exact. I went from a size 28 to a size 8, and I learned a lot along the way about myself, about others, and about the world in general. This book is a reflection on those lessons—and they aren't all what you might expect.

Let me warn you—this is no "How to Get Skinny Quick" guide. It's not a book about how I lost the weight and how you can too. Relax. You won't have to relive all the childhood trauma I faced or bear the brunt of my unhappy saga. This is a book about *shedding weight*—but probably a different type of weight than the type you're thinking.

Let me ask my original question a different way:

How much weight do you carry?

I don't mean those numbers reflected on the bathroom scale. I'm talking about the weight of pursuing perfection. As someone who has lost a monumental amount of weight, I'm familiar with the pressures women face to have perfect bodies and to *be* perfect in every area of life. I know what it's like to carry not only the weight of 336 pounds but also the weight of the perfectionistic ideal that has inscribed itself on our notions of femininity. And if I were to place a bet, I would guess that you, too, know just how cumbersome it is to carry the constant pressure of measuring up to the unspoken (and sometimes loudly spoken) body standards of the world around you.

I've had the opportunity to view the world from many different angles. The way others saw me as a size 28 is a lot different from the way they currently see me as a size 8. But you know what stayed the same throughout my entire weight journey? Me. At my very core. In fact, the way I saw myself in the mirror in plus-size clothes from Lane Bryant is no different from the way I see myself in that same mirror in my size 8 spandex leggings. Despite having reached the goal that so many people pushed me to achieve—whether through their bullying or their compassionate support—I felt no different. With so much weight gone, I still found myself waking up each morning, stripping off all my clothes, tiptoeing to the dreaded scale, and facing the stark reminder that I was still, even after all this hard work, *imperfect.*

So, you know what I did? I shed something else: my desire to be *perfect.* From those flabby arms to my cottage-cheese thighs that (still) rub together when I walk, I'm done with the pursuit of perfection. And I think you should be too. Because 336, 186, or 101—that number on the scale is not a barometer for your happiness. Or at least it doesn't need to be.

This book is about shedding the burden we carry because our bodies have a bit extra around the waistline, in that booty, or in those arms that we refuse to show off in a T-shirt. I know this book is for you because I know that I'm not alone in this journey. In fact, I think if we were honest with ourselves, we would all admit that no matter our size, we've been—or are—uncomfortable in our own skin.

Why should we spend our whole lives hating our bodies? Why should we feel anxious and uncomfortable when we're in a room full of people because we can't stop thinking about our muffin tops? What are we teaching our kids about their self-image? Why strive to live a healthy daily life only to be overly critical of our bodies every single day? Shouldn't we just be happy that we have bodies that live, move, and breathe? I asked myself these questions many, many times.

Faith is part of who I am. I always knew I was loved and valued by God, yet for years I struggled to let that truth sink deep enough to believe it every time I looked in the mirror. My faith has been my anchor in every area of my life, yet it hasn't been a quick fix when it comes to learning to love and accept myself. For years I spun in circles trying to figure out how I could possibly be this discontent after so much hard work. Eventually I stopped asking questions and started looking for answers. To find them, I had to let a few things go. So perhaps this book isn't really about shedding weight—it's about letting go.

- Letting go of the cycles of self-punishment for making normal human decisions, like eating a scoop of ice cream or an extra slice of pizza.
- Letting go of the constant anxiety we feel when we throw on a swimsuit that might reveal the scars and memories visibly written on our bodies from yesteryear.
- Letting go of the fear that our bodies are not good enough.
- Letting go of the idea of perfection; because the only woman I know who has a "perfect" body is Barbie, and she's made of plastic.

I believe that we are called to be the best, healthiest version of ourselves we can be; but I worry that the signals from the world around us are often crossed, leading us to believe that unless we *are the best*, we aren't worth much of anything at all. I worry that we're pursuing something that doesn't exist, and we are killing ourselves—both physically and emotionally—in the process.

I know I'm not alone. In our highly visual culture, we're reminded every day that our bodies don't fit the mold. Airbrushed beauties on magazine ads, perfectly proportionate mannequins in the mall, and flawlessly trim actresses all remind me how far from stunning I must be. We're hardwired to compare ourselves to others, and there's no way this Cellulite Cindy could ever compare to the Perfect Pattys and Stunning Susans all around me, right?

Right. And that's okay.

Because my goal is not to be Patty, Susan, Shanay, or Raquel—my goal is to be me.

In this book I want to talk about the good, the bad, and the ugly sides of weight, bodies, worth, and the pursuit of perfection. If my conversations with women across the country are any indicator, this is a topic that impacts all of us—all day, every day. Whether it's among the ladies in the small group I'm leading, through a commenter on my blog or within my Instagram community, or among the women listening with tears in their eyes while I share my story in an auditorium full of hopefuls, I have experienced firsthand the fact that my struggle is one shared by many. Nearly every woman I've had the pleasure of chatting with beyond surface-level banter— whether she's coming to me for help or is someone I aspire to emulate within my own healthy lifestyle—has expressed something she is dissatisfied with about her body.

We so often view our bodies as bad, imperfect, lacking, flawed, and in need of fixing. But what if we instead realized that our bodies are actually *good*? Bodies from every culture, background, and race. Bodies with disabilities. Bodies of every shape and size. All good. Right now, today, without changing anything at all. What would happen if we approached our body image with a sense of gratitude, compassion, and appreciation? Seems like a lofty goal, but stay with me. I want to help you learn to love *your good body* and see it as good—not as flawed or falling short. I want you to let go of self-criticism and lean into a fresh sense of body positivity.

I want to validate your struggle of being chained to the scale, and then I want to show you how to walk in freedom. Freedom from eating like a rabbit and freedom from being bound to junk food; freedom from feeling like you're torturing yourself with exercise and freedom from feeling too inadequate to start working out; freedom from wearing tainted glasses when you look in the mirror and from sucking in your stomach every time you see your reflection. You are free to pursue all aspects of health—physical, emotional, and spiritual—without feeling that you need to pursue someone else's version of perfection. You're free to find balance and set your own goals without being crushed by others' expectations. I want to help you see that you are free to love your body as it is right now, no matter what—even while you're moving toward better health.

Yes, my friend—there's a whole world of freedom out there for you to experience, and I hope that through my vulnerability about my journey to freedom, you'll feel empowered to pursue it on your own terms. Our goal is to find happiness *right where we are*, even if we're not where we want to be just yet.

> Our goal is to find happiness *right where we are*, even if we're not where we want to be just yet.

Throughout the book we'll look at ways we can progress on our health journeys. I'm not interested in telling you what to eat or what workout to follow, but I do want to help you find balance in all aspects of health. I want to help you change the way you think about your body, food, and exercise; figure out your right motivation; and learn to embrace who you are. Each chapter will highlight a step on the journey, and then I'll leave you with a quick action step and a question to consider.

Part of learning to love yourself as you are involves learning to speak to yourself with kindness and compassion. All too often we reinforce society's messages of perfection with the words we tell ourselves: "I feel so fat!" "I look awful!" "No one can love me like this." At the end of each chapter, you'll find a *flip the script* challenge where I've given you a new, positive message to say out loud and internalize. It's time we rewrite the lies we've allowed ourselves to believe about our bodies, replacing them instead with the *right* words, *right* framing, and *right* perspective.

One note: In this book we'll mention themes like diet culture, body dysmorphia, and disordered eating. If those are uncomfortable for you because of struggles you've experienced, know that I've been there too. Read through these sections slowly in a way that works for you.

So throw on your superwoman cape, girl—whether it's a size XS or a 4X. We've got a battle to win. As you make your way through this book, you're going to learn to stand up tall with your hands on your hips—no matter how wide they are—and your shoulders squared, shouting from the rooftops that you are choosing to love your good body as is while working to become the best possible version of yourself.

Grab another cup of coffee, honey; we're in for quite the conversation.

Chapter 1

BEYOND THE NUMBERS

If you think about it, all of life is built from numbers. Our big welcome into the world is preceded by nine months of anxious waiting. At about age one, we walk. At sixteen, we are granted permission to drive. At eighteen, around the time we land our first job, we're "permitted" to pay the government a cut of our income. At twenty-five, we can (finally) rent a car. At sixty-five, we're told it is time to retire. Somewhere between eighty and one hundred, on average, it's time to bid our humanity good day. And at 191 pounds, the whole world falls apart.

Or at least that's what you'd think if you were with me on that rainy Tuesday morning a few years ago.

As I shook off the remaining drops of my morning shower, I headed to my closet. Past the Christmas tree we store there. Past the suitcases. Past the boxes of baby clothes that I couldn't get rid of, even though my husband and I weren't planning to have more babies. Even past that *other* box of baby clothes (you know, *just in case*). There it was— the thing I had hidden like a shameful, dirty habit. In part, it was.

That scale had become my enemy numero uno. But like a long-lost cousin after you win the lottery, there it was, waiting for the attention it sought. Carrying it gingerly, as if it were a bomb, I soldiered back through the battleground, waging war in my mind as I tiptoed into the bathroom as quietly as possible and placed the scale on the cold, hard floor. And then, in that familiar choreography, I slowly lifted my legs one at a time and stood atop the twelve-by-twelve-inch square that had come to define my life.

My life has always been about the numbers—not just any numbers; *these* numbers. So when I saw "191" pop up on the cobalt screen of my digital scale, my mood quickly started to match that shade of blue. In and of itself, 191 is fine, just as 91 is fine for some and 291 is fine for others. But for me, that 191 couldn't be digested without a closely associated number: 336—the number I was at when I started my weight loss journey more than a decade ago. I'd lost so much weight, but keeping it off was a constant battle. I was up a few pounds from last week, and every gain made me worry that I was headed back to where I'd started.

Before I could even lift my somber head, I heard the feet behind me. There he was—my husband. And though my heart normally ticks up a notch when I see him, this time it sank into my stomach. How many times would he bear witness to my self-defeating square dance with that wretched metal scale?

Don't get it twisted—Phil is no fat shamer; in fact, he is just the opposite. Despite my ball-and-chain relationship with that scale, he has loved me throughout *all* the numbers: 336 (my highest), 169 (my lowest), and everywhere in between. For those of you who aren't quite sure the same is true in your relationship, don't worry—we'll get to that in a later chapter. But in that moment, supportive and loving as I knew my guy was, I couldn't think about his love. All I could think about were the rendezvous I'd had with other loves as of late.

That overly greasy, saturated-in-cheese slice of pepperoni pizza.

That massive burger paired with its favorite partner of all time: fries.

That decadent warm brownie topped with even more chocolate and served with a glass of whole milk (because dairy is a food group, don't you know?).

I tried to remind myself that life is about balance, but in that moment, there was no balance in my emotions as I went full-blown *teenage girl going through puberty who was just dumped by her new boyfriend of three days.* That number on the scale signified the end of my life, at least at that moment.

I'd been through this cycle so many times, yet each time those numbers served as a painful reminder of my humanity, my imperfection, and my shortcomings. Roller coasters are fun at an amusement park, but there's a reason the ride ends after only a few minutes—we can't handle the twists and turns too much longer than that. The roller coaster of my weight confirms that sometimes our bodies can prove to be too much. The 191 on the scale again reminded me that this ride was not yet over, despite how badly I wanted off.

I knew there was no quick fix. Those pesky pounds had crept onto my body with absolute ease, but getting them back off would be a tooth-and-nail battle. I knew they wouldn't melt off with a trendy fad diet, a quick jog, or the faulty promises of some magic pill. This would take work. A lot of really diligent work.

As the drops of water from my shower finished evaporating into the air, I rehydrated my skin with the moisture of a good salty cry. And that's when Phil could no longer keep silent.

"Why do you do this to yourself, babe?" he asked, his genuine empathy coupled with the memory of a thousand times we'd had this same conversation. He'd just as soon throw the scale in the dumpster and never look back.

Knowing that there was no way he could possibly understand, I snatched that scale up again—this time with some force—and I marched back to my closet, past the Christmas tree (no sugar cookies for me this year) and those boxes of baby clothes (I'll be darned if I'm going to *willingly* gain weight again!). I shoved the scale as far back into its dusty home as I could, pushing the surrounding boxes tight against it, as if to figuratively starve it of any fresh air and show it who was boss. "I'll be back for you," I threatened aloud. But it already knew . . . we'd meet again soon for our normal affair. Same time, same place, same routine.

In the familiar pattern that had come to define my life, I put one foot in front of the other, dried my tears, and moved on with my day. I reminded myself of the numbers—five hours until lunch (a healthy one, I promised myself), eight hours until my husband would be home from work (plenty of time to plan out how I was going to attack these pounds), and just sixteen until I could go to bed and put this horrible day behind me. Yet again.

THE NEVER-ENDING REMINDER

Most of us find the weight of the world overwhelming to carry at times. For me, the *world of weight* is even heavier. For years it defined my whole existence. Although I had been carrying *more than* the normal share of body fat for as long as I could remember, others always saw me as something *less than*. That's the toughest part of carrying extra weight. I own—and quite like—my curvy girl status. But we all know that this isn't just about

> Although I had been carrying *more than* the normal share of body fat for as long as I could remember, others always saw me as something *less than*.

being curvy. And try as society does these days to celebrate bodies of different shapes and sizes, we all know that it often falls short. Bodies that don't quite meet the thin ideal are often briefly showcased and then tossed aside, replaced again with more of the same old, same old that we've come to accept as the perfect standard. This preoccupation with thinness is so routine that it's almost become unspoken, yet it's something that women face their entire lives.

My first exposure to this came in kindergarten through a boy—let's call him Nick. He was a nice-enough brown-haired kid who seemed to always wear the exact same pair of knee-high socks and khaki shorts. Still, what I remember isn't his niceness but a passing comment he made to me while playing. Nick felt it was his duty to let me know that my face was "different." "It's funny . . . your cheeks look like this," he said, puckering his lips together and pooching out his cheeks. "You look like a chipmunk!" And just like that, five-year-old me instantly became self-conscious about having a round face.

I'm sure Nick didn't do the same to you (if he did—gosh, that kid really gets around). But I'd imagine you have an experience of this variety somewhere in your past too. Those words spoken to us in our childhoods often play a formative role in our personal growth throughout our lives. The weight of those words lingered with me, intensifying at an alarming rate until it peaked in middle school—perhaps the toughest time in any young girl's life. As I bounced around the country between my divorced parents (moving around thirty-two times before the age of eighteen), the other kids, who barely had time to get to know me, often met my *weight* before they met me. Thankfully, bullying is taken quite a bit more seriously these days, but around that time it was often dismissed under the "kids will be kids" mindset. Kids will be kids; and as it turns out, kids will also be *little jerks* if you let them. The bullying was relentless.

Over and over again, year after year, from kindergarten until I graduated high school, it seemed like *everyone* felt entitled to draw attention to my weight. They'd tell me I needed to go on a diet or assure me that I could lose the weight if I really wanted to. If I had a cold, strep throat, or a broken finger, my doctor's first suggestion was always to lose the weight. At church I felt the sting of the youth leader's message when he highlighted how the Bible instructed us to "take care of our temples"[1] (so mine was a megachurch . . . big deal). Whether the words were outright and bold or presented in the guise of compassionate care, I carried them all the same way. They were a heavy burden on top of what crept up to 336 pounds by the time I entered high school. What began as growing up in poverty and having limited food options eventually led to poor eating habits, which then ultimately paved the way for using food to soothe an aching soul.

For years I carried a body in excess of 300 pounds and maintained that weight until I lost it in my adult years. And all throughout, those words followed me. Truthfully, I could probably fill the pages of this book with stories about how mean kids in school were about my weight. It was excruciating. The ridicule cut deep, almost as if the comments were tattooed onto my psyche.

I think these types of memories have such an impact because they happen so early for many of us. I'll always remember walking into Ms. Garden's class, where the chairs were scattered around the room in no particular arrangement. We could choose the seat we wanted every day as long as we got to class and claimed it before anyone else did. You remember that game, right? It was like an old-school mashup of musical chairs and *The Bachelorette*. Yet, like most of those extra-tanned, one-note men who show up determined to snag the grand prize, I was regularly reminded that *I was not the one*.

Our sixth-grade bachelorette? Sheila. She was perfectly popular in every way. Most girls flocked to her with unbridled determination to touch the hem of her ~~garment~~ skort. I avoided her at all costs. But I'll always remember the day when I showed up late to Ms. Garden's class and found that the only available seat was right in front of Sheila. As I maneuvered my body into that row and sat down, I felt my hips hang over the side of that front-and-center chair. The familiar and comfortable sound of mindless chatter filled the air as I breathed a sigh of relief that I had avoided being made fun of . . . for now. Then I heard it out loud—a voice cutting through the silence: "Who here thinks that she should wear bigger clothes?"

Pause.

Who? I wondered. Then I realized.

"She needs clothes that actually fit," Sheila opined, sounding authentically nauseated that I dare wear clothes over my body. "You can see her fat rolls through her shirt!" And then the chorus started—not a chorus directed by the hands of Ms. Garden but the chorus of a song that followed me throughout my early years: corporate laughter speckled with the shame, disgust, and pity that all comprised the song of my life.

I'd been in situations like this before. Sometimes I got up quietly and left; sometimes I tried the art of the comeback (not my greatest strength, but darn it, I tried). Sometimes I pretended that I hadn't heard. But that day, I just sat there and counted the numbers . . . again.

Only 46 more minutes until this class will be over. Two more years until I'll be done with middle school. Six more until I'll graduate from high school. Just 714 miles from here to the cute little town in Tennessee we visited when I was younger where I'll escape to one day. Just 160 pounds to lose and I won't be fat anymore.

The theater of my teenage life was quite melancholy. I cried. A lot. I internalized even more. By the time I graduated high school, my soul bore the marks of my physical experience. I had no self-esteem, no support system, no rest from the torment. I'd come home from school each day and barricade myself in my room, lie in my bed, and cry. And like a sad story on repeat, this came to define my daily life.

RESOUNDING SIGNALS

Don't stop reading yet. This book is no somber sonnet or boo-hoo brochure about my life. In fact, this book isn't even really about me. I'm merely sharing my stories in hopes that you'll take the time to reflect back on yours. This journey is about so much more than recognizing who we're *not* and how we don't measure up. It's about going through a process of learning to celebrate who we *are*. It's about taking a good look in the mirror and watching a smile form at the corners of our lips. It's about feeling our fingertips graze the curvy hills of our tummies and beginning to love every inch. This is about learning the lyrics of an anthem of freedom and dancing like nobody's watching—even if *everyone's* watching. That's why we start here. People *are* watching, so perhaps we need to stop waiting to enjoy ourselves and our bodies until they stop looking. They never will—and that's okay.

I'm about to make a shocking statement. Are you ready?

Women are so hard on themselves.

We know this already, right? We're expected to be a size 2 but cook like an Iron Chef. We're expected to keep the house clean, tend to the children, keep a steady stream of income, and meet all of society's (unrealistic) ideals of feminine per-fection. We have social media feeds to keep fresh, friends to impress, and a whole slew of fellow women to prove our adequacy to. (Side note: Friends you have to impress aren't true friends.) The demands are real. And true to our nature, we often internalize most of the pressure. We take it upon ourselves to police our own actions and make constant corrections to ensure we meet or exceed all the standards set before us.

And can we be honest? It is utterly, completely, almost beyond description *exhausting*. Lest you think this is just the ranting of a bitter woman, let me assure you it isn't. I love being a woman. In fact, being a wife, a daughter, and a mother are among the gifts that I cherish the most. But those aren't the areas of my life that get me down; it's the areas in which that old message—*I am not enough*—gets reinforced.

We're often reminded that the grass is *not* always greener on the other side. Yet over and over again *green, green* grass is dangled in front of our faces. Companies have mastered the messaging that catches our attention and reveals a need we didn't know we even had. Just think of the magnificent magazine promises that taunt us as we check out in the grocery store:

"Be a size 2 by summer!"

"141 ways to tone up those problem areas."

"Eat better, stress less, and drop 10 pounds with this simple trick!"

"Tear your fat, ugly face off and put it in the trash because you'll never be anything unless you drop 25 pounds."

> We're subconsciously conditioned to believe that who we are at our core is never actually enough.

Okay, so I'm exaggerating on the last one, but you're familiar with the rhetoric that drives us to look in the mirror and quickly turn our heads away in disgust. We're subconsciously conditioned to believe that *who we are at our core* is never actually enough. We're told that with some small change, act, or purchase, we can get one step closer to perfection—a perfection that is temporal, fleeting, and (spoiler alert) can never actually be attained. But the problem here is that the image we're striving for isn't presented as "perfection." It's presented as "normal," and it is dangerous territory when we come to understand *perfect* as *normal.*

Since so many resounding messages about our supposed shortcomings center around numbers, it's no surprise that we tend to reduce ourselves down to one thing: the number on the scale. We let our weight, jean size, or the millimeters of thigh gap we wish we had become the most important thing to us—the thing that defines who we are and what we're worth.

Some astounding numbers also undergird the bait and switch of the self-improvement industry. According to McKinsey & Company, the global beauty industry generates $500 billion in sales a year.[2] Yes, billion. Each year. That's larger than the economies of many industrialized countries in the world. And most of that profit comes because of the subtle reminders sent our way that something isn't quite right with us.

It's no wonder, then, that we become discontent with ourselves, feeling like we're never enough. Because the very thing we're reaching for is forever just beyond our grasp—always available with the next product, with the next diet, or at the next size down. We're always looking at the grass on the other side of our circumstances, forgetting the simple truth that the greenest grass is the grass that gets watered.

So, let's water our grass, shall we? It might be easy to think that my argument here is that we should run far away from industry standards of beauty—grow our hair out, stop shaving, and let the acne pile up on our faces after eating so much we've got the meat sweats (unless that's your thing—in which case, you do you, girl). No. This is about finding balance and loving who we are while also working on who we are.

Nothing in life is ever invented and perfected at the same time. We think nothing of buying the latest and greatest Apple product, only to receive an update a few short months later to "fix" the errors that came with the device when we bought it. We're used to buying flawed products, yet we've somehow fallen into the trap of believing that when it comes to us, it's an all-or-nothing game—perfect or bust. What if we could learn to love ourselves and improve ourselves at the same time? What if we took back control of the narrative and, instead of letting a multibillion-dollar industry or the voices of our past tell us who we should be, we penned our own stories? What if we saw ourselves as more than a number and learned to see our bodies as good?

The resounding messages in our heads can scream loud enough to knock us off track. So before that happens, let's get a few things straight. You do not have to travel down the road of feeling less than. Of loathing what you see in the mirror. Of allowing the numbers to jumble up your day and send you into a cycle of crash dieting. With careful planning, the right map, and some intentionality, you can turn away from Self-Defeat Lane and onto Self-Love Boulevard.

That's what this book is about. This is about reprogramming our GPS so that no matter where the roads of life take us, we can find our way back to the people we were meant to be. We're "fearfully and wonderfully made," as Psalm 139:14 (NIV) tells us. That second half—wonderfully made—is easy to cite but unfortunately quite easy to forget. What about the first half? What does it mean to be "fearfully" made? The Hebrew word that scholars translate as *fearfully* is *yare*, which means "to stand in awe of" or to "be afraid."[3] To me, that says there's something just a little scary about our design. There's something in us that should be feared. We are full, multidimensional beings with unique personalities, quirks, likes, and dislikes. When we reduce ourselves to a number, we erase so much of ourselves. Maybe that's the true starting point in any health journey. How different would our approach be if it came from a place of realizing our value and wanting to change the way we think about and treat our bodies to reflect that truth? If we knew how to tap into the magnificent power and potential given to us by design, we'd approach the world with such a confidence and drive that people would say, "Watch out! She is fierce. And here she comes!"

I invite you to reprogram your GPS with me throughout

these next few chapters. Let's take a long drive together and chat about what makes us unique, what makes us tick, and what stands in the way of our living our best lives. We'll talk about being confident in our relationships and saying no to comparison. We'll look at how we can have healthier relationships with food, the scale, and movement, and how we can continue our health journeys while viewing our bodies as good vessels that we can celebrate, not broken vessels we have to fix. Don't worry—I'll drive. And as I do, I'll let my guard down. I'm going to show and tell a lot about me. Much of it will not be flattering. But as you get to know me, I hope that you'll reorient yourself with *you*. I hope you will learn to love your good body and treat it with compassion.

We'll take it slow here, not zero to sixty in ten seconds flat. We'll enjoy the scenery and many different types of terrain, because I truly believe this message is for all of us, despite our vast diversity of lived experience. Together, we'll camp out in the trenches where things are hard and wake up early to enjoy the sunrise. We'll laugh together, cry together, and bare the depths of our souls. Then we'll stare victory right in the face with the confidence that comes only once we learn to love ourselves as is.

That brings us right to our first step in changing the narrative and learning to accept our bodies as good. Pause and look at the *flip the script* statement on the next page. If this lie is one you tell yourself, how can you replace it with the truth? Reflect and take action!

Flip the Script

Instead of telling yourself, "I'm nothing but a number," say this instead: **"I'm so much more than a number."**

Reflect

How would your life and attitude change if you could believe that you are enough—not after some self-improvement projects, but now, just as you are? What would help you believe this?

Action Step

Take a minute to jot down some of your personal attributes. What do you like about yourself, and what makes you *you*? Are you friendly, kind, hardworking, smart? Can you sing, cook, paint, organize, lead, teach? What about your body? List some things you like about it. No negativity allowed!

Chapter 2

PERFECTLY IMPERFECT

For years, *perfection* in my mind was a direct reflection of what the entire universe had been drilling into my head since, well . . . always: *There's too much of you; you need to take up less space.* I would have done pretty much anything to get small enough that the world would finally think my presence mattered. Strange, isn't it? We live in a world where bigger is always better, until it isn't.

Chasing perfection is a fundamental aspect of life—and while it can sometimes drive us toward excellence, more often it becomes a goal that we obsess over but can never attain. How much are we willing to give up to attain what we think of as the perfect body?

In my years of striving for skinny, I traded a lot to try to make that happen. I'll never forget a particularly ridiculous diet I was on for a few months. It was so strict that I ate nothing but slivers of lean meat, bland slices of roasted radishes (and other vegetables of the *disgusting* variety), and an apple or orange. I was absolutely starving, all the time, yet I'd turn down every treat presented to me. Special cupcakes in the breakroom, delicious lunches my boss brought in, and even my beloved coffee—gone. I was so committed that I moved heaven and earth in a stressful season of life to precook chicken and steam broccoli and take them to the big family get-together we were having at my sister's house. Family members from all over the country were there to visit, and the excitement of reunion filled the air alongside the smell of burgers and brats. And there I sat, next to Phil and my toddler daughter, eating dry chicken and tasteless broccoli. For what?

Those trade-offs defined a lot of my life. I declined invitations for fun trips with friends, dinner parties, travel weekends, and birthday parties, all because I thought I'd never be "just right" until I was as small as I could be. Forget the s'mores around the campfire or the ice cream late at night (or any time of day, really). I had to get smaller. At any cost. No time to stop and smell the ~~roses~~ hot dogs cooking on the grill.

That same pursuit of perfection will get you, too. You needn't be a health expert to know that the type of eating I described above is unhealthy and probably fits the definition of disordered eating. And *disordered* is a great term because so much of my life was *out of order.* I was pursuing a number in hopes that it would make me healthy. Now, though, I pursue being healthy and what comes with it. Number be darned.

Don't get me wrong, there *are* trade-offs when it comes to pursuing a healthy lifestyle. I can't honestly tell you that you can just hope for the best and it will all work out. All *good* things require effort, and health is a good thing. But when the effort becomes our only focus, something isn't right. We're out of alignment.

This is a call to pursue balance—because pursuing perfection is a dead-end street. In many ways, our quest for perfection is killing us.

THE COST OF CHASING PERFECTION

Recent statistics show that most Americans report feeling unhappy with their bodies—a full 79 percent of us, including men.[1] Alarmingly, this number grows to 91 percent when you look at women alone.[2] What's more, just 5 percent of the female population naturally possesses a body that looks like the "perfect" body commonly portrayed in the media.[3] That means if you throw one hundred women in a room, ninety-one would have their heads between their knees because of the way that five or fewer in that room looked. So many of us are made to feel left out because our bodies fail to conform to a standard we think everyone is supposed to meet.

For many women, obsession with weight and bodily perfection starts early. By just age nine, somewhere between

50 and 80 percent of girls identify a desire to lose weight.[4] And get this—nearly 40 percent of fourth-grade girls diet![5] This number grows in middle school, again in high school, and again in college, when body-related concerns take an especially dark turn. Full-blown eating disorders (that is, eating disorders that go on to define lengthy periods of a person's life) often develop in the college years. More than thirty million people in the United States suffer from an eating disorder,[6] and eating disorders have the highest mortality rate of any mental illness.[7] Every sixty-two minutes, at least one person dies as a direct result from an eating disorder.[8,9]

Maybe this isn't your particular struggle. But it isn't disordered eating, per se, that I'm caught up on when I read these statistics. What I walk away with is a simple yet harrowing truth: Women are so obsessed with attaining the perfect body that they'll sacrifice anything, even their own health and well-being, to get it.

But what's the perfect body? Who gets to decide what *perfect* actually is?

We each have our own fantasized version of what would make our bodies perfect. We set out to tweak this or change that, only to find that once we do, yet another "necessary" improvement pops up almost immediately. What's perfect? A six-pack or curves? Bigger boobs or smaller ones? Being fifty pounds lighter or having defined muscles lining our upper arms? It's quite the loaded question.

Yet here I am—asking you. What is it?

Close your eyes and visualize the "perfect body." Isn't it

interesting that we only think about how this body looks? Most people don't think of the perfect body as one that is "perfectly capable of running a 10K" or "perfectly able to lift an impressive amount of weight." Those are things that the perfect body is able to *do* in many people's minds, but it isn't what the perfect body *is*.

Though your visual understanding of a perfect body is likely to vary based on your culture, your own body, and your exposure to different types of media, most representations of perfect bodies meet three basic standards. Perfect bodies are:

- **Trim. Not too skinny, but certainly not too *not* skinny.** Women with curves are shown more and more in mainstream media, but they are still often isolated to specific brands or types of products. When is the last time you saw a plus-size woman in a jewelry ad, for example? For the most part, women are expected to have curves—but only in all the right feminine places and only in the right amount. Not boulders. To be fair, our sisters who might be underweight by mainstream standards also get a lot of grief for their perfectly normal bodies. Women are expected to be thin and curvy. Too many curves? Gross. Too few? Also gross. How in the world do we even begin to satisfy the critics?
- **Nimble, agile, and flexible.** The purpose of a body is to carry out body-related tasks—moving, eating, breathing, processing. Inherently human *stuff*. But

you wouldn't know it by looking at the visuals of
perfect bodies. Though we all carry different abilities,
limitations, and health histories, the most celebrated
bodies are those that are free to live life without
constraints. That isn't the case for everyone, and our
conversation needs to acknowledge that.

- **Aesthetically pleasing to others.** Perfect bodies are
those that acknowledge, reflect, and embody mainstream ideas of beauty. These aesthetic standards are
nearly impossible for all of us to achieve. If you're
a woman of color, you might have it even worse
because on top of these unrealistic standards, you're
often asked to align so many other elements of your
identity. Perfect bodies are those that don't go against
the norm.

Most of us couldn't attain the "perfect" body even if we
wanted to. We're too tall, too short, too "big-boned" (Do
bones really vary in size? Asking for a friend . . .), too skinny,
too curvy, too athletic. We have imperfect skin, hair, or
makeup skills. We might have physical limitations or a cultural background that's not appreciated. But the truth is, having the "perfect" body is not the only way to be beautiful. And
beyond that, overinflating the value of having the "perfect"
body diminishes the gifts, skills, and talents that are inside of
us waiting to be awakened and shared with the world.

Trying to chase body perfection is harmful, but there is also
a sacred imperative for not wanting to uphold mainstream

beauty standards. These standards reinforce so many poor habits—greed, jealousy, comparison, self-centeredness, and beyond. That *fearfully and wonderfully made* thing we talked about earlier? It's sort of hard to uphold that as a core value when we're trying to break out of our own make to drive a different model. You were not intended to be the product of an assembly line with a uniform recipe that guarantees no deficiencies. Your body is the carrier of your story; your story is the carrier of your purpose. So let this be a reminder that though pursuing health, fitness, and even a body you're comfortable in can be a fine pursuit, it should never get in the way of your greater mission and purpose in life. Your body is incredible and should be celebrated (we'll expound on that later). But there is *more to you* than your body.

> Your body is incredible and should be celebrated. But there is *more to you* than your body.

Focusing on perfection has a way of causing us to miss out. I've given up a lot in my own pursuit of whatever body priority I had in any given season of my life. At times I've even eaten so little all through the day that I had a massive migraine by afternoon. I've refused to hit the gym because I was afraid of what people might think of me when I was fumbling around trying to figure out the machines. I am convicted when I think of potential moments lost—moments with connection, meaning, purpose, and love—because of my preoccupation with being the smallest size possible.

This body obsession defines the journey of womanhood for all of us, and it comes with a cost.

A 2017 study found that women spend an average of $313 per month on their appearances, including cosmetics, skin care, haircuts, manicures, gym memberships, and other fitness costs. That adds up to $3,756 per year, or $225,360 over a lifetime! Imagine what else we could do with that money.[10]

The costs are not just financial. The most rewarding aspects of life and womanhood are those things that money can't buy and beauty can't enhance. How much *time* goes into this pursuit of physical perfection? How much *anxiety* do we build over our bodies? What moments of life are we missing out on because we're too busy worrying about what the mirror has to say about us? Of the four in five women who report low body esteem, nearly all (89 percent) have reported avoiding important activities like hanging out with friends and family, participating in activities outside of the house, and going certain places because of some insecurity they have about their bodies.[11]

This hits me right between the eyes. Why? Because I've been that person. I have two kids—my daughter, Kennedy, who is nine, and my son, Moses, who is six—and I've recently faced the sobering fact that not only do they not care about the size of the jeans I bought last weekend, but also my obsession with these minor details is taking away from some of the major memories I need to be focused on making. I've been too worried to take my kids for ice cream, not because sugar is bad for *them*, but because of what it might do to *me*.

At times I avoided taking them to some of the world's most beautiful beaches—a mere few miles from our house during the five years we lived in Florida—because I was worried about how others would perceive me in even the most modest of swimsuits. I was too busy trying to attain perfection, and I was missing out on the good life right in front of me.

UNLESS

As a society, our obsession with perfection (and not just body perfection) is on an upward trajectory. At first glance, this might seem like a good thing. After all, what could be wrong with trying to better ourselves? Isn't that what our design equips us to do? Well, yes. And also no.

We are biologically and psychologically designed to reach for the stars and be the best version of ourselves we can be. However, even at its most illustrious stage, that best version of ourselves varies based on our unique story. We've got battle scars that tell the tale of us no one else can tell. Those scars shouldn't be hidden—they should be borne to the world as a testament of our strength, resilience, and individuality. The wound that lingers on my left knee from crashing my bike when I was ~~little~~ young (I was never little) equipped me to teach my children how to get back up again after a fall. Relocating thirty times before I turned eighteen was difficult and unsettling, but that cluster of experiences led to my ability to connect with people quickly and adjust to change more readily. Battle scars are to be appreciated. Yet we hide them, afraid that their presence highlights our imperfections and renders us less worthwhile than those who seem to have no battle wounds of their own.

The pursuit of perfection can have a significantly negative impact on our mental and social well-being. Perfectionism has been defined as "a combination of excessively high personal standards and overly critical self-evaluations."[12] In our pursuit of perfection, we set unrealistic expectations for others and, more importantly, for ourselves. We tell ourselves that we'll never be anything, never amount to anything, never achieve unless . . .

And that *unless* is very individual. Of course, this book is about chasing bodily notions of perfection, but we know that the *unless* that taunts us can take a variety of different shapes and forms. That *unless* polices our actions and is causing us to fall apart. Thomas Curran, a psychologist known for his work on perfectionism, notes that "in order for us to compete, we need to know where we stand, and to know where we stand, we need to know our attributes. That tends to breed a lot of social anxiety, upward social comparison, and we, as a consequence, worry about how we look to other people."[13]

Sound familiar? Much of our anxiety comes because we've locked ourselves in a personal prison of perfection and given the key to other people—our ex-boyfriends, our childhood nemeses, our well-meaning but tactless aunts and uncles, the mean girl in our homeroom. The funny thing about this is that those people don't even know they hold your key. And what's even funnier is that you don't need to ask their permission to take that key back. You—yes, you—can take back control over this narrative. You can unlock the prison of perfection. You can set yourself free and flip the script.

You don't have to be perfect.

In fact, you can't be perfect. You know who's perfect? Barbie—but she's plastic and shoved in a box. You know who isn't perfect? This girl. And she's a lot more interesting than Barbie (I promise, I will stop throwing Barbie under the bus in this book). Sure, she's got some extra baggage—a few pounds to lose, loose skin, and the same bags and wrinkles that plague most women. She's got stretch marks—a testament to the human life she carried inside her. She's loose in places she wishes she was tight and round in places she wants to be square. But she's unique. She's valuable. And she has a lot to offer the world.

I can't tell you that I don't ever think about my insecurities. I can't tell you that I don't still shed a tear from time to time when my jeans are tighter than they used to be or when I try on a shirt in my size that, as it turns out, is *not* actually my size. And I can't tell you that I don't sometimes still obsess over nutrition and exercise (things I've genuinely come to enjoy). But I can tell you that I've learned to let my scars show more and more. You may see a before-and-after weight-loss snapshot, but if you look a little closer, you'll see the cellulite, loose skin, wrinkles, and muffin top in the after photo.

What good would it do to make people believe that this whole weight-loss journey of mine was no less than a magic trick? I want to share the reality that it hasn't always been rainbows and butterflies. Losing the weight didn't render me a body that automatically grants me contentment or happiness or satisfaction. There have been highs and lows and many different trails through which I've had the "opportunity" to walk this thing out. I want people to realize that. That's why I've learned to wear my battle wounds proudly. I've learned to let that fat show freely. I've learned that I'm not perfect and I don't want to be. I've learned to love myself at every size. I've learned to love myself while also working on becoming the best version of myself.

This process doesn't happen right away. It can't. The cultural coding that wires us to be self-critical and pursue perfection in the first place has etched itself deeply on our psychological makeup. This coding didn't happen overnight, so we must allow ourselves the grace, space, and time needed to rewrite that script. But it can be done.

> I've learned that I'm not perfect and I don't want to be. I've learned to love myself at every size.

Maybe perfection isn't the goal. Maybe the goal is seeing our bodies as truly, wholly good and knowing that good is better than perfect. When we give up perfection as our goal, we don't have to prove ourselves to anyone else, nor do we have to live up to their expectations.

Throughout this book, we'll learn how. But before we do, I want to share a bit more about how I ~~got there~~ am getting there.

Flip the Script

Instead of telling yourself, "I'll never be perfect," say this instead: **"Perfection is not my goal. I am uniquely beautiful exactly as I am today."**

Reflect

What are some scars from your past that have contributed to the person you are today? What has pursuing perfection cost you?

Action Step

Grab a pen and sketch your idea of the perfect body. Label the things that you think make it "perfect." Then ask yourself why those things make it perfect and what value those "perfect" attributes actually add to the world around you.

Chapter 3

YOU GET TO TAKE UP SPACE

There's a common saying that you shouldn't judge someone until you've walked a mile in their shoes. I have often thought we might understand others better if we walked a mile in their *jeans* instead. I spent so much of my life wondering—sometimes aloud to those around me—what it would be like to be, to feel, and to look like *her*. And *her*. And *her*. And *them*.

Shy is not a word that describes me nowadays. But as a kid, I was alarmingly quiet. Though many simply chalked this up to my personality, I now understand that it was because there was so much going on in my head that I had no residual energy to use on speaking. I expended all my effort on presenting the best version of myself to the world.

I can now laugh at how naive I was to think that the right color sweater or the right name-brand jeans might overwrite someone's feelings about a body I held deep insecurity about. Still, I knew I had to try because the weight I carried on my shoulders—not my thighs—was such a burden. I can still feel that visceral pain of being crushed by a stranger's judgmental glance or the laughter of others who saw only my weight—not me.

I spent most of my life feeling like I took up too much physical space in the world. In my twenties, I began "fixing" that problem by making myself smaller. But even then I realized I was still afraid to take up space in people's lives, so I deliberately began to push against that mindset. That's a big part of the reason why as an adult, I've never met a stranger. If you so much as smile at me in the grocery store, I'm for sure going to pause and ask you about your day, your life aspirations, or your family pet. But a major reason I've figured out who I am is because I remember who I was, the pain I experienced, and the struggle I faced to feel like I had something to offer the world.

I've often wondered what it must be like to be *on the other end* of that pain. While I'll never know, perhaps it might be helpful to share my experiences. So, let's talk about being fat. But before we do, let me clarify—I use the word "fat" intentionally, not in a denigrating way. I use the term here because I want you to feel the experiences of it—experiences that are largely negative because of the fat stigma that pervades society.[1]

As a woman who has been a myriad of sizes, I have to note that it is quite uncomfortable to be fat—not necessarily physically. I think most people want to hear about those physical burdens of carrying extra weight. The backaches, the leg pain, the mobility limitations—all the things we've come to characterize as consequences of being larger than "normal" (and please don't get me started on that designation). That's not what I want to emphasize here because physical limitations can happen as a consequence of a variety of life factors. And honestly, conversations like that are often unproductive. To critics, they prove a point that is incomplete ("See, it's uncomfortable to be fat. You should try this diet so you don't have to feel that way!"). To those who are unhappy with their own weight, they serve as an unhealthy barometer ("I'm big, but not that big"), reinforcing the comparison trap. And to others, they merely stir up pity, which might be well-intentioned but is misplaced.

I think it's healthy to reflect on feelings of being fat and how they can radically change some of our moments from joyful or neutral to downright terrible. Take flying, for instance. What should be an everyday normal human routine can quickly turn into a harrowing experience when you have to ask a flight attendant for a seatbelt extension on an airplane. Then there are the awful glares you get when a passenger finds out *you're* the one sitting next to them. Your legs are so big they spill over into the seat next to you if you don't clench them together tightly through the duration of the flight. That same clenching happens with your arms, which become blobs of disgust to most people they accidently graze, so you bring your elbows into your ribs, making yourself as small as possible. That's both to avoid the inconvenience of sitting next to another person while fat and also to try to make yourself unnoticeable. *There's* where the pain comes in—your muscles get sore and tired from what is effectively a solid core workout. Your back hurts. Heaven forbid you fall asleep to pass the time because perhaps your body will forget that it is being punished on this two-hour-and-forty-seven-minute flight. So you get to sit with that physical *and* emotional pain for the entire duration as you are forcibly reminded to ponder your excess.

Amusement parks are quite similar. What should be spaces of carefree fun can become a carnival of nightmares when you're large. That might sound like an exaggeration, but if you've ever been pulled off a ride by a park employee because the seat belt wouldn't close or had to watch friends and family *on* the rides while you waited from afar because of size limitations, you know it isn't. Eventually, the embarrassment proves too much for many of us. I could likely count on two hands the number of day trips to amusement parks that I've turned down simply because I couldn't bear being reminded of my body all day during what should have been a release from the cares of normal life.

It isn't just the fun stuff that brings pain when you're fat. Professional settings—even those that you might think would uphold the utmost principles of human dignity—also carry a significant fat bias. In the years leading up to my weight loss, there were certainly a few fat-phobic comments made in the workplace. Luckily, there were far fewer bullies surrounding me day to day than in high school. But when I thought I was finally free from harsh criticisms, it hit even harder when out of nowhere another snarky remark popped up and blew an airhorn in my ear.

Every decision I made—big or small—was preceded by the question about how my fat would factor in. If I was carpooling on a youth group trip, I'd think about how to negotiate the front seat. I was torn because I didn't want to seem selfish or call attention to myself, but I was nervous about what would happen if I had to squeeze in the back seat. If my dad invited me to join him on an adventurous snowmobile ride during one of my trips to see him, I'd worry about how my body might take up too much space or slow down the vehicle. If I went out to eat at a restaurant, I was concerned about ordering the wrong thing—the kind of menu item that might give the server or nosy people around me the satisfaction of a mental *I told you so.* They might think, *No wonder she's fat. Look at what she's eating!* often while eating the same plate of chicken fingers and fries that I'd ordered. Nearly every single time I walked in a room, I anticipated who might already have judged my worth, my contributions, and my personality based on my size.

> Nearly every single time I walked in a room, I anticipated who might already have judged my worth, my contributions, and my personality based on my size.

This is the burden of being fat: not the fat itself but the weight of others and their unsolicited opinions, stares, and input on what diet, exercise program, or magic pill might "fix" you. When you're fat, you are seen as fundamentally broken, and soon you start to believe that about yourself. Thus, you do anything and everything to not acknowledge the weight, in hopes that you might be able to enjoy a few fleeting moments of peace. What this does, though, is constantly reinforce the idea of weight in your head. It's like telling someone to look at a bowl of M&M's but *not* focus on the green ones. Try as hard as they might to ignore the green ones, they're still going to find them.

This was the story of my childhood and young adult years. So many conversations avoided. So many nights out foregone. So many activities abandoned. My voice was basically nonexistent back then; and it wasn't because my vocal cords were broken. I hid—mostly from others but also a bit from myself—to find reprieve. By the time I reached the later years of high school, I was so wounded inwardly and so self-conscious that even though I craved connection, I stopped making the effort to be a meaningful presence among others. My back still slumps from the way I'd walk the hallways of the building with my head down. To this day, I can still physically feel the anxiety that comes with simultaneously being the biggest body in the room and the least valuable to others. I truly believed that a body this size had no business occupying space with its ideas, its thoughts, its hopes, its dreams, or even its awkward teenage energy and naiveté. I came to believe that I was so fat that the world had no use for me.

ROCK BOTTOM

Rock bottom is one of the darkest places we can ever find ourselves. The thing about rock bottom, though, is that it isn't an easily identifiable location. Some moments in my life as a big woman were defined by laughter, joy, friendship, and success. And then at other times it seemed like I was trudging through mud. Just like climbing the stairs, navigating life at that size took the wind out of me. In those moments, it was hard *not* to see all of my struggles as a consequence of my size; after all, every anxiety in my life before then had always been a by-product of my fatness. So when life threw all it had at me, I felt extra hopeless. Not only did my problems seem insurmountable, but I also felt like I wasn't even worth the effort to dig myself out of the pit.

After high school I moved to Virginia, found a small apartment where I lived on my own, and took a job at a little bookstore in town. As thankful as I was to have a job, it barely paid the bills. Most times, after I covered rent and other necessities I was left with less than twenty dollars to stretch across two weeks until I'd get paid again. When something unexpected happened—like needing a new tire or a doctor's appointment—I was hanging on to hope and a prayer that somehow the money would come just when I needed it to. By my mid-twenties as a fat girl living paycheck to paycheck, I found myself at some complicated intersections.

Depression set in. Hard. I think we all tread these waters a time or two in our lifetimes. We keep our heads above water, but no one can tread water forever. Eventually our legs and arms tire. Do we give up and throw in the towel? Do we keep going, hoping that the lifeline we so desperately need is on the way? These questions brought me to a crossroads that came to define the rest of my life thus far.

As I returned home from work one night, I remember descending the stairs into my tiny, rundown apartment. With each step, I felt my body rise and fall, a somber metaphor for my mood as of late. As a young woman struggling to create the life I wanted, I had experienced several waves of panic about my choices, my history, and my future. I walked into my cold apartment and took a good look around. In that moment, I saw several suitcases in my mind's eye— metaphorical baggage overflowing with the measures of my weight that held me back. One was full of pressure—pressure on my joints, back, and knees. Another large suitcase carried the past. It held agonizing words spewed at me from peers in high school, looks of pity and disgust from strangers on the street, and even the well-meaning but misguided "advice" that seemed to come at social gatherings and even doctor appointments. The third bag was the most cumbersome to me; it held a thousand tries and fails at losing the weight.

That night was no different than most. There were no extenuating circumstances, no extraordinary stressors looming over me. Yet that day, the baggage I'd held for years was suddenly heavier than ever. Somehow, the weight of the world hit me full force that wintry evening. It felt so cold, not just outside but in the world I was navigating. I could barely stumble into my room before letting out what was without a doubt the most gut-wrenching sorrow I had ever carried in my body. I allowed myself to free-fall backward onto my bed, not even totally sure whether I would land on the mattress or the floor. I threw one hand over my eyes and left one leg hanging off the bed. And I sobbed. I anguished. I angered. I labored.

And I surrendered. I had been trying for my entire life to hold it together, hope and pray I could fix my "weight issue," and move on to be who everyone wanted me to become. But as I lay there with warm tears pouring down the sides of my temples, I surrendered to painful memories that filled nearly every single day of my past.

Like the needle from a tattoo gun, I felt the physical etchings of every hurtful word that had ever been hurled at me. A photo album of my life began to play through my mind—me with a fake smile in a swimsuit, me tugging at my sweater to conceal my belly, or me standing behind everyone in a group picture to hide as much of my body as possible. Sweat began to pour from my skin as I felt a level of physical anxiety I had never experienced before. The moisture from my body—both the sweat and the tears—saturated my sheets. I was drowning, not in water but in sorrow. With a grit and anger that my timidity would never allow in social settings, I uttered a whisper through the breathless tears. Simple, meaningful, sober:

"I can't do this anymore."

IN THE MORNING, WE WAKE UP

We live in a culture that loves to focus on *can*. "You can do it!" seems to be an ever-popular mantra. We say it even when we don't mean it. And as a lifelong optimist, I believe in the value of speaking positive words as we interact with the world around us. But perhaps we don't spend enough time legitimizing the *can'ts*. In my rock-bottom moment, there was no greater truth for me than the words I spoke: I could not do it anymore. I didn't need to hear that I could lose the weight or that I would get through. I needed to be okay with resting in the fact that the present reality could not sustain me.

When I woke the next morning, the sun crept through my windows as it always had. And with almost the same level of shame as I suspect you'd get from a hangover, I lifted my heavy body—coat still intact—out of my bed and walked through the living room into the kitchen. *Here we go again.* I looked at the SlimFast in my refrigerator, knowing that I needed to refuel my body to embrace yet another inevitably difficult day of navigating the world around me. *Or,* I thought, *I could just head to the deli next door and grab a bacon, egg, and cheese biscuit.* I almost couldn't believe that after an entire night of crying every tear I had to offer, I wasn't getting a Cinderella moment. No fairy godmother had come to turn my pumpkin of a body into princess material. Instead, I woke up the same 336-pound girl I went to bed as, sobered but unchanged.

I'm not sure I knew it at the time, but I truly believe that that morning and the evening that preceded it were do-or-die moments for me. I cannot express the depth of sorrow and anguish I felt, and I could not have gone on that way. And so, I believe it was a miracle that morning when I looked atop my refrigerator and beheld a brown package that had been collecting dust for some time. My curiosity got the best of me as I grabbed hold of it and dusted it off, pulling out several starter books for a popular nutrition plan that had taken the United States by storm at that time. (I find it important to note that it wasn't an overly restrictive diet plan. Though my understanding of the complexity of weight management wasn't as mature then as it is now, I already knew that severely restricting my food wasn't the key to long-term success.) As I flipped through the first few pages, I remembered when I'd shoved the books away several months prior because they looked so similar to everything else I had tried—and failed at—in the last decade. I closed the books yet again—and then reopened them. *Okay, well, I might as well try something. Let's do this today.*

That moment—sitting in the kitchen on a sobering Saturday morning still in the clothes I had worn the evening before—propelled my entire weight-loss journey. Really, it looked a lot like many moments before. There was no special circumstance, no magic pill, no choir of friends who had banded together to convince me that I could do it, and no excessive determination magically funneled into my body. That ever-absent fairy godmother hadn't slipped in and sprinkled me with skinny dust. The only difference between that day and all the others in the previous two decades was the excessive amount of desperation that had wrecked me and brought me, quite literally, to my knees.

That desperation helped give me purpose. I was desperate enough to start taking a closer look at my relationship with food, how I was approaching exercise, and what was driving my feelings of complete hopelessness. I was desperate enough to stop believing the lie that I couldn't take steps toward becoming my healthiest self; that desperation fueled the confidence I needed to do this for *me*, not for anyone else. I was also desperate enough to stop buying into the false notion that I was a 336-pound woman and nothing else; I knew I had worth, even if those around me couldn't see it. I'm not sure my mind fully grasped in that moment what the next few years would hold for me, but one thing's for certain: It knew I was desperate. And desperate people are willing to do desperate things.

THE DRIVE OF DESPERATION

We'll talk more about my wellness journey in the following chapters, but my focus here is less on the *how* and more on the *why*. After all, everyone can tell you how they do what they do; it's the why that really drives things home in our everyday lives. Our why has everything to do with what motivates us to make changes and how our motivation impacts what happens next. And what happens when our primary motivation is desperation?

I know it's a lot easier to write this as someone who is now *not* 336 pounds. I'm fully aware of the privilege that comes with writing about health, wellness, weight, and weight loss as someone who can often slip through the world without the soul-crushing hypervisibility of an overweight individual. But time makes us wiser and bolder. Over a couple of years, two times of gaining and losing pregnancy weight, and lots of trying and failing, desperation took me from 336 pounds to 169. In that respect it succeeded. But it didn't stop there. When my weight crept back up from 169 to 199, it was desperation again that took the reins in my journey from 199 to 174. And the story goes on . . .

Desperation is a driver, but it isn't always a good one. It can get us from point A to point B, but our lives aren't linear. They are full of complex intersections, detours, and different terrain that desperation can't handle. Desperation was a catalyst for me and an important one; I'm thankful that it was there when I needed it. But desperation has also wrecked a lot of my life.

Desperation isn't like an Uber driver; you can't exactly finish your ride and bid it good day. It likes to hang around. So even when you arrive at your destination, desperation is often right there with you, anxious to hop back in the driver's seat and take you somewhere else. When you pack on five pounds of holiday weight or stress-eat when your kids experience problems, desperation picks up the keys and drives you a little further in your journey of self-loathing. When joy supersedes sorrow and you let go (even just a little) of your nutrition or fitness habits, desperation doesn't always party with you; it reminds you where you came from and is happy to drive you further into obsession and anxiety.

By definition, desperation involves a state of despair. It requires you to be so unhappy with current conditions that you engage in change, even if that change is rash or extreme.

When we resort to desperation as the primary driver for our health, we are seeing ourselves and our worth as only the sum totality of our bodies. We assume that if we're this miserable at this size or shape or (insert any other body anxiety here), *surely* we'll be happy and content when we address that issue. We despair about those characteristics, and we often obsess about them. We cringe at the photo of our frenemy on Instagram who has her six-pack abs on display and then automatically remember how our own midsection doesn't measure up. We hear someone talk about getting healthy or losing weight and we become paralyzed by anxious feelings of never being able to attain that for ourselves.

When desperation drives our change, it's often a telltale sign that the change we're seeking might not be for us. Desperation often comes when we recognize that we aren't living up to some social standard or some commonly accepted way of being, and we feel compelled to change because of external pressure. That's ultimately far less motivating than a decision we make for ourselves. So though desperation might work, it might not be the best way to bring about the most successful transformation.

For me, desperation led to recklessness of the variety I'm

trying to speak to in this book: self-destruction. Negative self-talk, particularly, was a familiar friend through those desperate times after I'd hit rock bottom.

- *You'll never be anything but a fat girl.*
- *You'll never land a man; who would want you? Who could find you attractive?*
- *You're more likely to die of a heart attack than you are to actually make a change. No change has ever stuck before. What makes you think this time will be different?*

Desperation can drive deep, dark thoughts, the recklessness of which can drive dark and toxic behaviors. For instance, a lot of eating is driven by feeling. That's why Thanksgiving holds such a special place in our hearts (no one *really* likes dried-out turkey all that much). When you become reckless with your words, you can quickly become reckless with your eating. For some of us, that means bingeing—eating to take the negative feelings away. For others, it's restrictive eating—punishing ourselves for being fat.

Desperation is a hard one to shake. A small dose can drive healthy and effective change, but a lifelong habit can create miserable cycles of defeat.

As I reflect back on that tear-filled evening of desperation that launched my weight loss, I recognize that I latched on to the *wrong* feeling and allowed it to propel me forward. In that moment, I replayed every hurtful comment, every judgmental gaze, and every moment of body-related trauma.

I let the negative energy of those moments drive my action when I could have done something so simple yet so radically different. I could have *loved* myself enough—without any asterisks or clauses or conditions—to change.

DIG DEEPER

One of the most prominent components of successful, lasting change is motivation. We know that the more time we spend working toward something, the higher our probability of success. That's simple, right? Stick with something long enough, and you're bound to succeed! But it isn't quite that easy. In and of itself, time has no power; it is a neutral agent that exists in the world for us to use. A clock on the wall has no power unless we *give* it power. Putting in the time isn't enough; we've also got to put our feet on the ground and begin walking out a life of purpose, moving forward with a clear vision of what lies ahead. Our motivations, our drivers, our goals—our *whys*—are the primary catalysts by which we succeed. When we lose sight of our why, we lose our focus and, often, our identity. We repeatedly find ourselves back where we started from because we forget that journeys are not just about time—they are about effort, energy, and motivation.

We all have moments when we're so desperate for change that we are willing to do just about anything to get there. We sacrifice and, in some cases, torture ourselves because we so badly want change. We want a quick fix, so we find something that works within a short amount of time. I've tried this a million times over. I've tried taking hormone injection shots that promised quick, lasting weight loss. I gulped SlimFast like water. I purchased a total body exercise machine. I wanted change fast. But that's just it—I wanted *change*. In and of itself, change isn't a healthy goal. Change is ambiguous and an ever-moving goalpost.

Many of us with body anxiety just want to change our bodies and, if we drill down, we might not have a good reason. Sure, we spout off the things we're supposed to say: "I want to be healthier!" or "I want to live longer for my kids." Is that what it's *really* about, though? What does that next-size-down little black dress you saved in the back of your closet have to do with living longer for your kids? Our desire for change isn't just about that—I know it and you know it. It may be a component, sure, but it certainly isn't the totality of our motivation. We've got to be a bit more honest, checking our real reasons and motivations.

If you want to be healthy—really healthy, apart from some pseudo standard of body reflection—you need something more, something authentic. You need to find your *why* and ensure that it is healthy, realistic, appropriate, and personally meaningful. This is the single most necessary tool to have in our back pockets as we embark on our long-term journey toward health. We've got to recognize that time doesn't have value here; this isn't a *six-weeks-to-skinny* plan, nor is it one where we tap out after five years. The goal isn't a quick fix, and it isn't to be a certain size within a certain time frame. The goal is bigger than weight loss, fitness, or our end results.

It's to learn that we can pursue wellness and see our bodies as good at the same time.

When we're determining our true why, we need to dig deep. We can't resort to a cute slogan or mantra that *should* motivate us. We have to think about what truly drives us to make changes—while also learning to practice compassion toward our current selves.

- What will pull you off the couch when you absolutely do not feel like moving your body? And also, what will pull you to stay on the couch when your body is honestly telling you that it simply doesn't have what it takes today?
- What will make the healthy and balanced dinner choice when you're weighing the options after a long day? And what will also give you the permission you need to order pizza because you know that small indulgences from time to time are not only acceptable but healthy?
- What will motivate you to look in the mirror and choose compassion toward yourself when your expectations of yourself don't match reality? And how will you celebrate—in a healthy way—when you experience the results of your hard work on your body?

Surface-level motives will absolutely not cut it when we're toiling in the land of these nuances. Desperation may give

you a big dose of adrenaline
to start some new habits, but
it will not sustain you over
the long haul. And a motivation that sustains us over time
is what we want. No matter
what our ultimate health goals

> Desperation may give you a big dose of adrenaline to start some new habits, but it will not sustain you over the long haul.

are, we want to make changes that are drenched in self-love
and reflect our understanding that our bodies aren't just
bodies—they are agents to carry out our greater calling and
purpose in life. We must embrace the process and align our
desires and motives with that calling.

Let's talk about a few characteristics of a good, solid why.

Your why is not about being skinny

I support a health-at-every-size philosophy and believe that it
takes movement and intentionality at every size to be healthy
and well. So, as someone who has made this mistake in the
past and still fights it almost every day, I want to clarify that
your why is not, cannot, and should not be about being
skinny. Being thin is not only an unsustainable why, it is one
that is closely correlated to disordered eating and a host of
other behaviors that run afoul of health and wellness.

Will you get skinny by being healthy? I think that answer
depends on who you ask. If you ask me, I'll tell you no.
Because at 336, skinny is 250. At 250, skinny is 170. At 170,
skinny is 145. And it goes on and on.

So let's just toss this goal away, shall we? You can be skinny and healthy. You can be skinny and unhealthy. You won't often find me using the term *overweight* because that term assumes there's some magic number that defines our total health, which is, to be frank, ridiculous. What the scale tells you is for you and your doctor. That's it. How you perceive that number is entirely up to you. But I beg you—don't let skinny ever, *ever* be your why. Let your why be about something that isn't as fleeting as a number on the scale or a dress size.

Your why shifts over time

As much as I decry skinny as a primary goal, I have to recognize that my goal was exactly that for many years. I wrongfully assumed that being "skinny" was the only way to measure up to what I thought everyone was expecting of me. And I would venture that for many of you reading this, it was—or even *is*—your why too. That doesn't make you some monster fat-shamer, nor does it invalidate your efforts to be intentionally healthy and well. If that's your why right now, it can pave the way to a deeper and more sustainable motivation as you learn what's most important to you in your wellness journey.

One of the reasons I sought to write this book was because time has given me so many opportunities to renew my focus and reevaluate my own journey. I recognize that my why has changed many times over the years. At first my why came from a sense of desperation. Then it was wrapped up in this notion of proving to others that I could lose the weight. Next, it was about proving to myself that I could do it. Eventually it truly became about health and quality of life. Throughout my adult life, my why has ebbed and flowed, changed and shifted. I believe you should give yourself permission to change yours, too.

Life is always changing, and so are our commitments, goals, and priorities. That's why skinny as a goal doesn't work well. Honestly, sometimes skinny just doesn't "fit" with where life takes us. But if we find the right why, health will fit with us no matter where we go. If we're getting healthy for the right reasons, our why will move with us throughout the ups and downs of life. Being flexible and forgiving enough with ourselves to let parts of our why go and to allow new parts of it to join us on our way helps us truly focus on lifelong health and wellness.

Your why solidifies your commitment

While today I have a more balanced approach to wellness, it wasn't always that way. For years I was tempted to try anything and everything if it meant there was the slightest possibility of edging that slider toward the left on the scale. I'd pay large amounts of money (if I had it at the moment) for anything that claimed it would be my golden ticket to reaching my ultimate size goal. Even now the temptations still arise. A friend does a smoothie cleanse and tells me all about it, and my first instinct is to give it a try. I get back from a vacation and feel bloated and fluffy, and I consider eating like a rabbit for a few days.

But having a deeper why solidifies the commitment I've

made to choosing wellness over frenzy in my health journey. It keeps me from jumping ship and doing something crazy based on the direction the wind is blowing. My why runs so deep that it doesn't just push me to "get skinny," but it consistently nudges me toward rejecting the pressures of diet culture and instead walking toward feeling well both inwardly and outwardly.

Finding your why will help you in the long run by giving you a reason to "tap out" of any incoming diet and exercise fads that promise quick results but require no long-term commitment. When you set a why that is focused on lasting health and wellness—not dropping weight at any cost—you'll quickly realize that those fads are a waste of time and an incredible waste of money. Why not focus on lasting change instead?

When you find your why, you won't be apt to jump on some new bandwagon because the quick fixes promised by that bandwagon don't fit with your overall goals. After all, you've now determined something that matters to you for the long haul. When you identify what that is, your level of commitment is solidified. This process becomes more personal and thus much more real and doable. You're in control here, and because you call the shots, you can be serious about meeting your goals because they honor your ultimate commitment.

Your why sustains you

How often do you get in your car, turn the keys to start your engine, and then sit back and say, "All right, where should we go?" Probably never, right? There's an old saying that when the going gets tough, the tough gets going. But the tough doesn't just set out on any old journey—it gets going somewhere specific! That saying is all about action. When life gets you down, do something different to keep moving forward. When we're struggling, we might not even know how to put one foot in front of the other. Life has a way of throwing things our way—jobs lost, relationships dissolved, health deteriorated. In those moments, it's easy to let ourselves go. I'm not talking about going a day without makeup or gaining some weight from stress-eating during a global pandemic. I'm talking about forgetting that we are the authors of our own stories. As women, we often feel that it is our responsibility to tend to everyone else around us. We're charged with supporting our spouses, tending to our kids, cooking, cleaning, and caring, but in the midst of life—just regular life, not even *hard* life—we forget to care for ourselves. By finding our why, we can set ourselves up for a life that's more fulfilling.

When you put in enough time to find your why and you've etched that why into the depths of your heart and mind, you're already a step ahead of most people. For many, the moment the desperation wears off, so, too, does their entire why. Identifying in your heart a set of reasons that drives your action can help ensure that you are constantly self-reflecting and tending to you. We've been tricked into thinking that self-care is selfish. Let me—and thousands of counselors, researchers, psychologists, and mental health professionals—assure you: it isn't. And this isn't just a secular concept. The Creator created you with human limits and free will; he also took a rest during Creation. You've got just one life to live. Finding your why can help you live out that life to its full potential, throughout all of the many seasons.

Your why is specific to you

I've learned over time that my body is and should be unlike anyone else's.

Try as hard as we might, humans don't fit as neatly into boxes as we wish we did. So I've stopped letting my journey be defined by those around me. I've got physical, emotional, and mental challenges and strengths that are different from anyone else's. I know that your why might not allow you to eat cake, but listen—this girl loves cake, and your journey does not have to define mine. I can sit and admire you as you run a marathon or do CrossFit—but I'm not feeling it right now so I'm gonna skip it. Just as your methods and my methods for healthy living might not be the same, so, too, might our whys be different.

Honestly, I'm still calibrating my why. Some days I swear it's that I want to be the best me I can be. I want to have a sharp mind and a quick body. I want to program myself to do the best I can at everything I do. Other days I have to admit that my why walks a fine line between "I want to *be* comfortable in my own skin" and "I want to *look like* I'm comfortable in my own skin." Desperation has never fully left my side, and we're still working on some stuff. Often my why involves some feeble attempt to rewrite the past. I think about the hurtful words spoken to me, and I like to think of every moment of movement or act of diligence as one giant "proved you wrong" to the haters of my past.

My why began as a desire to prove to myself that I had what it took and that I could do it, even if my whole life had been defined by the crowd of voices that told me I couldn't. I'm over those losers now. Today, my why is about my family—my husband and two kids. My why keeps me accountable for ensuring that all aspects of my wellness journey are healthy and balanced. I want my daughter to grow up different from me. I don't want the why that defines her—the thing that drives every move she makes and every breath she takes—to be about her weight, her size, or some artificial standards of perfection. I want her why to be all about her. I want her to smile for the camera and not think at all about rolls or extra chins. I want her to free-fall onto her bed every single evening out of a sense of wonder and appreciation for life, not out of desperation to change who she is or what she looks like. I want her why—the catalyst for all that she does in life—to be about radical self-love and acceptance, no matter how she aligns to society standards. I want her to learn to love her body and know that it is good, without exception.

So, for me, for now, my why is that too. My why is about freedom from self-doubt. My why centers around the notion that I am enough as I am, and I want to continue to rest in that. My why is about radical self-acceptance and self-love, acknowledging that in order for my purpose to be accomplished, I have to love myself through the process.

What about you? What's that thing that reaches you at your very core and tugs you to move forward in love rather than in desperation? Call me crazy, but I have a feeling there's a piece of you that longs for the freedom to take up space in this world without worrying that you're taking up too much space. Let that longing motivate you. Ask yourself what it would feel like to have a why that has nothing to do with what size or shape your body is. Then let that why push you toward freely caring for your body with no surface-level strings attached.

Flip the Script

Instead of telling yourself, "I want to change my body because I hate the way it looks," say this instead: **"I can make good health choices out of love, not hate."**

Reflect

What would it look like if your drive for better health was based on overall wellness and loving your body, rather than pressure to lose weight? In what ways would the journey be more enjoyable if the starting point was love and not hate?

Action Step

Jot down your why and post it somewhere you'll see it often, like on your bathroom mirror, in your planner, or as the wallpaper on your phone. It may change a bit as you ponder it, but this gives you a starting point for digging deeper as you go along.

Chapter 4

THE STARK NAKED TRUTH

Since I introduced my kids in the last chapter, I suppose I should spend some time here unpacking what is an oft-unconsidered but monumentally important element of health and wellness journeys: romance. And just a note for those of you who find yourselves a bit more . . . puritanical . . . than others: This chapter acknowledges the existence of a certain human activity between two married (and fat) adults. It's sex. And you've been warned.

But let's start with some basics. My marriage has always been one of my top motivators in life. Even though my own parents were divorced and had a complicated dynamic when I was growing up, I do know what full love and support look like, and the hope of developing and nurturing my own future marriage was a primary driver for many of my decisions in early adulthood. As I worked through the trauma of my past, though, I had a hard time believing that a family would ever *be* my reality. I felt unlovable and questioned whether anyone would ever be attracted to a woman of my size. In my mind, any unrequited crush meant that I was too big and not appealing to the eyes of the guys.

Dating while fat can be complicated. Sort of like there's a tiny but enthusiastic market for, oh, I don't know . . . headbands? Miatas? So, too, is there a certain level of enthusiasm for bigger women in the dating marketplace. The problem? It's weird there. I can recount several dates where I wondered why the men I was with had chosen to go on a date with me. I soon found out: It was physical. And though these were FINE, UPSTANDING CHRISTIAN MEN™, it didn't negate that their intentions were less than . . . holy.

I'm no man-hater, but I do need to note that my most profound movement toward health came when I swore off dating for a season. When I wasn't looking for value in the eyes of others, it turned out that I could really focus on the things that matter. And then, boom. A year or two later I met the most awkward punk rock boy you could ever meet: my (now) husband, Phil.

Phil is the penultimate professional, wise beyond his years, cuter than he probably should be, and the smartest and most self-sacrificing man I've ever known. But the first time we met, I remember breathing a huge sigh of relief and thinking, *Whew. Okay, thank God. At least there's not going to be any awkward romantic tension.*

It was a few years after my rock-bottom moment, and I was working and attending college full-time. Phil and I were both music majors with just about one more year until we'd have our undergraduate degrees in hand. Just before he ditched music to pursue a career in communications, Phil made a pretty penny accompanying vocal music majors like me on the piano. (While I didn't love being in the spotlight, I'd spent my entire life in front of people singing solos and with choirs—mostly because people asked me to and I didn't want to tell them no. I had zero desire to assert myself into any all-eyes-on-me situations, so I just closed my eyes and opened my mouth to sing while pretending that there wasn't an entire room full of people looking at me.) My vocal coach recommended him, and though I had no idea who that Phil Wagner guy was, I knew I had to lock in an accompanist. I emailed him that same day, and we arranged a time to meet.

At the time, I was a hyper-professional career woman, and I arrived wearing dress slacks, a flowy blouse, and pointy-toed flats. Phil walked in with black spiky hair, a nose ring, ripped jeans, and a hoodie. Based on our appearances, we weren't just apples and oranges. We were like apples and hairspray (Phil's hairspray, probably). Though I knew for sure I wanted to be married to the man of my dreams one day, I was content being a single professional and working on becoming my best self. By the looks of things, Phil was content crowd surfing at punk shows and being the life of the party.

That seeming mismatch was a real bummer because as it turned out, Phil was such a nice guy. We'd meet regularly to practice for upcoming recitals, and each time I got to know him a bit better. He made me feel like I hadn't before. One day he saw me running in from work to get to my vocal lesson, and without a wink, he said, "Jen Taylor, can I carry your books for you?" I melted. In a sense, that small gesture made me feel accepted and worth someone's time and effort. And no one could make me laugh like Phil. At the end of each semester, vocal majors were required to perform our pieces for faculty judges as a final exam. The waiting room was always packed with nervous students waiting for their turn, and all the practice rooms were filled to the brim with people making last-minute preparations. There was one piano in the middle of the waiting room, but it was sort of an unspoken rule that no one could touch it. Phil, knowing no fear and always able to schmooze his way out of any real trouble, snagged it and told me to start singing. I was caught off guard, not wanting to be embarrassed if we got into trouble. But Phil had a plan. "If anyone comes over, Jen Taylor, just bow your head and pretend like we're praying. It takes a real jerk to interrupt someone who's praying." That was Phil—always a lighthearted bundle of energy.

Except he started to mess with my heart. We quickly became friends, and that grew and grew into a life-altering companionship that gives me hope on my worst days. Time has a way of changing people. I dropped my hyper-professionalism and learned the value of a good pair of jeans. Phil dropped the nose ring and mohawk (actually, all of his hair). Our stereotypical styles changed; our love only grew. We got engaged and set a wedding date just a short ten months later on an autumn day in the heart of Central Virginia. We had a beautiful ceremony, officiated by our pastors and followed by a fun time surrounded by friends, family, and loved ones. We danced the night away, ate too much cake, and loved celebrating the love we had for each other.

But then came the wedding night. For those of you raised like us in the church, you know that the wedding night is sort of a *big thing*. It's that moment where your relationship is official in the eyes of God and the law. And once the county courthouse receives certification that you're officially hitched, you automatically receive your official "do it" pass. The one that gives you permission to do, you know . . . *it*.

If you're someone who has struggled with weight and body image your whole life, you know just standing in front of the mirror naked by yourself can be its own form of trauma. Though Phil and I were quite excited to have our "do it" pass in hand, I failed to account for the fact that in order to *do it*, I'd need to take my clothes off. Like—all of them. I'd shaved my legs, waxed my chin beard, and accounted for not having an unplanned pregnancy on my wedding night. Yet in the hustle and bustle of the wedding day, I totally forgot that your wedding evening wasn't the time to revert back to your muumuu and fuzzy slippers.

Phil, the consummate gentleman and quite the mind reader, knew that something was up. And perhaps he had the wedding night jitters too. Because we sort of just laughed awkwardly while looking dead in each other's eyes. And I'll never forget hearing what were by far the sexiest words to ever fall out of my husband's mouth: "Um . . . do you just want to go get chicken fingers or something?"

And so we did. Wedding clothes and all, we walked down the block from our tiny hotel and got greasy food. We talked, laughed, and planned for our future. We held hands as we walked around the stone streets of our little downtown area, and then we went right back to our hotel room and promptly fell asleep. Before we did, we spoke our I love yous to each other, and I'll never forget Phil's words: "I think you're the most beautiful woman alive." When you're a plus-sized woman who has spent her whole life in fear of intimacy and vulnerability with others, no more meaningful words can ever be spoken. I'll spare you the details, but let's just say those words permeated the evening air and gave us plenty of, um . . . food for thought . . . when we finally got around to consummating the marriage the next morning.

We have to be honest with ourselves, ladies. Sexuality is a fundamental element of humanity, and having and enjoying sex is built into our design. The problem, though, is that we're often too wrapped up in our own insecurities to really get to that place, even with those we love. I was in the middle of a weight-loss plateau when my husband and I got married. I had already dropped 100 pounds, but love came and did its thing, and I had gained a bit of that back before walking down the aisle. That alone didn't bother me. But the thought of baring my whole naked body to another human—willingly?!

I suspect that many of you reading this haven't fully gotten past this either. Perhaps you're just dipping your toe into the dating world and thinking about intimacy that lies ahead one day down the road. Or perhaps you've been married for a while, but the tides of life have brought a little more fluff around your midsection. Either way, it is incredibly difficult to heed the advice that we laid out in the first few chapters. You know, the part where we agreed that we weren't going to pursue the "perfect" body or worry about what other people thought about our bodies? Well, that's hard when sex is so inherently visual!

The principles we outlined earlier do still apply. Even in your sexual relationship with your spouse, I believe it is absolutely critical to love your body, imperfections and all. There are a myriad of reasons why, and those reasons hold true no matter how your significant other sees your body.

My husband and I have chatted long and hard about men's perspectives on women's bodies, and we've come to agree that there are a couple of different perspectives that men tend to have on the subject.

NEUTRAL NATE

Believe it or not, Phil (who went on to get a PhD in communications and is now a professor himself) has a lot to say about body image. Because he has battled his own weight monster throughout his life, questions about how we view our bodies are regularly a part of his thinking. We are both infinitely curious about why our bodies matter so much to us, and we talk about bodies all the time. We talk about bodies in motion, bodies in sports, bodies in the grocery store, bodies and how they eat, bodies in bed.

Though I doubted him early on, over the past twelve years, Phil has proven that he loves me ~~despite~~ and my body. For the first few times I got undressed around him, I was so . . . modest. I'd cover the areas you were supposed to cover, making sure my towel or robe was appropriately seductive but not traumatizing. And that's what I thought my body was: traumatizing. I couldn't comprehend that someone would find me attractive. I gradually let my guard—and my towel—down, expecting to catch a look of disgust on Phil's face. And I waited, and I watched. And it never came. To this day, I still at times find myself not believing it when he calls me beautiful or lingers with his eyes.

After a few years of marriage, and many miles into my weight transformation journey, I finally worked up the courage to ask Phil a tough question but one I needed to know the answer to. I walked in the living room, where he was sitting on the couch, and asked, "Do you really find me attractive, or do you just pretend so you won't hurt my feelings?"

I expected him to turn off the TV, ask me to sit beside him, look deep in my eyes, and either tell me that it was time for me to hit the gym *or* that he loved me perfectly the way I was.

That didn't happen.

He looked up at me, rolled his eyes with more force than I'd seen before, and said, "That's such a stupid question." And then he went back to doing what he was doing.

I didn't know whether to be offended that he didn't foster my desire for approval or happy that at least he wasn't disgusted by me. But I realized that part of his response was based in his own lifelong weight struggle. Phil wasn't even planning on dating anyone before I came along. For one, he was focused on finishing college and building his career. But on a more personal note, Phil was insecure about his body, just like I was. He had been bullied about his weight since he was very young, and while he didn't let that keep him from running after his life ambitions, he, too, questioned whether a lifelong partner would ever find him attractive.

Over the years, as we've both worked on our bodies and our health, losing a combined 300 pounds, we've both become body-positive crusaders. He celebrates my curves, and I genuinely believe he loves them. But we talk about the older days when my vulnerabilities ran a bit higher, and he swears that men don't care what our bodies look like.

I know, right? Eye-rolling. Absolutely positively untrue.

But maybe it isn't. Maybe, just maybe, he's right. Research backs this up. A recent article debunks the ever-pervasive idea that men are only attracted to skinny women.[1] In the study, more than 2,000 male and female participants were asked to rate the body size and attractiveness of images of fashion models—and then to estimate how the opposite gender would rate the images. Both men and women overestimated just how ideal the other gender would find thinness and attractiveness. And you might have guessed that the result was strongest in women. Women consistently thought their thin bodies mattered way more than they actually did to men. So . . . breathe.

Attraction is real and important, but attraction isn't tied solely to the body. It also involves personality, sense of humor, connection, and a multitude of character qualities. I absolutely refuse to believe that by some base default, men care only about the size of our thighs, waists, or breasts. That's not fair to men, and I don't believe it is true. I believe many men have the emotional depth and capacity to love despite there being fat, cellulite, wrinkles, or saggy skin on a body.

Each relationship is different. Might the visual aspects of the body be a real issue in a relationship? Perhaps. But maybe it isn't just men being pigs; women also have hang-ups. When we can't get over our own hang-ups, might we be pushing them off on men? I mean, men have those hang-ups too. Talk to a man about his insecurities, and he'll often cite the size of his wallet, his muscles, or his reproductive organs as a genuine point of concern. That's why those things are the subjects of so many jokes in the media. And really, ladies— is that all you married your man for? Or if you're single, is that all you're looking for? No! Your ability to snag a well-financed, well-endowed meathead is not synonymous with your happiness. You're looking for a partner in crime; a spiritual connection; someone with whom you can build a family and a legacy. A lover. A friend. Perhaps we need to give men the benefit of the doubt that they're looking for the same.

How many dates have you put off because you're afraid of one day having to get naked? How many opportunities have you foregone because you're afraid that they'll lead to a reminder of your imperfect body? Maybe all men aren't Body-Positive Bobbys who think you're beautiful at any weight, but maybe many are Neutral Nates—those who don't notice or care what your weight is.

PETE THE PIG

Giving men the benefit of the doubt is not only critical, I think it's only fair. But we also know that some men— certainly not all men—are so inherently focused on the visual that it creates a catch-22 for those of us working to love ourselves as we are. Not all women have the luxury of a supportive husband who loves them no matter their size or the number on the scale.

There are a variety of reasons for this, many of which

have less to do with men themselves and more to do with the objectifying images of women we see all around us. While size diversity is becoming more mainstream, our culture still often upholds the thin ideal—perhaps especially in contexts of romance. Female sexuality is all too easily associated with a certain body type, one that many of us don't have and never will.

We need to be honest and note that some men are fundamentally flawed in their thinking. If your significant other is not the body-positive advocate you hope him to be, know that you are not alone. I know women who have bounced from diet to diet like a Plinko chip because they keep trying to land their husband's approval. I know others who put on a good front but have cried to me about their husband's "passing comments" or "jokes" about the extra they hold around their midsection (particularly after birthing children), comments they want to brush off but can't. And yes, I know women whose husbands have outright made demands that they lose weight or modify their bodies in some way.

Let me be clear: This is not normal in a loving relationship. At best, it's naive and ignorant. But that's not a call to abandon all. Relationships take work and communication. Talking about your body can be healing and important to your own confidence and view of self. Regardless of whether or not your husband is supportive of your weight and size, learning how to verbalize your thoughts on the matter can breed a new level of intimacy. Whether with a Neutral Nate,

Pete the Pig, your therapist, or your best friend, here are some tools to help you get the words out.

Clarify your expectations—for yourself. As easy as it might be to brush it under the rug, let's all just own an uncomfortable truth: So much about our body journey can become about crafting a body *for others.* We think we should lose weight so we can be more attractive to our husbands or potential dates. We choose our health goals based on what we think our romantic partners want us to be. That's not healthy, even in an intimate relationship. First and foremost, remind yourself that your body is not a reward for anyone else. It doesn't exist merely to bring visual or sexual pleasure to another person. Instead, it's a vehicle for you to live life, walk out your purpose, and enjoy the process of it all. Your primary goal is to shape your health and wellness so your body is equipped to carry you on that journey.

Bodies are handcrafted to navigate us through life. Celebrating them is appropriate; celebrating them *together* with your spouse in an intimate way is appropriate—and fun. But even in those settings, your body does not derive its value from other people, even those you love most intimately. Your sexiest self is your healthiest self, both inwardly and outwardly, so decide for yourself what makes you feel sexy and beautiful. Pursue those goals because they're something you want, not because you're trying to fit someone else's ideal.

Change your thinking about *thinking*. Remove the self-doubt you have about your body as a sexual agent. Sex is one of God's greatest designs, and it needn't be something it wasn't designed to be. It's about unity—two individuals coming together in their full vulnerability. Letting our guard down to that degree is what makes it such a sacred act . . . and what makes it fun. The width and weight of your body are not what make getting frisky so amazing. In a sense, reducing sex to being good only if your body looks a certain way is stripping away the depth of intimacy you could be experiencing with the one you love. It may sound crazy to some, but when Phil grabs my love handles and pulls me close and kisses me like he's going off to war, it is the biggest turn-on. Not just because he's a great kisser, but because his hands can travel across the surfaces that have caused me the most angst throughout my entire life. Now *that's* intimacy. Just as baring your sacred secrets brings you closer to a friend, baring your skin to your husband can do the same. Let your guard down a bit, and be willing to get vulnerable. Chances are, the things that you're so discontent with bear no real weight in terms of how attracted your husband is to you. If you haven't found the one yet, now is a great time to shed the self-doubt you have about that future encounter too! And to be honest, it's the love and companionship that make sex something special— not some arbitrary body standard.

> Reducing sex to being good only if your body looks a certain way is stripping away the depth of intimacy you could be experiencing with the one you love.

Talk about bodies. You want your husband to care about

the parts of your body journey that are important to you, so communicate that to him. I remember so many times becoming frustrated with Phil over just how much he *didn't* seem to care about my body. Sure, I could appreciate that I could be the size of a straw or the size of a hippopotamus and he would still find me attractive, but sometimes a girl wants to chat, you know? He loved me for me, he said—I never believed him. So eventually, we talked about it.

It took quite a bit of open communication for me to help my husband understand that I wanted him to care about my body.

Not too much.

Oh, and not too little!

Oh, and not like that!

But that's what it's about. Open, honest, vulnerable communication. The same holds true for men who are a bit less forgiving in their view on bodies. Although it is difficult, we owe it to ourselves and to our relationship to be honest about how those comments make us feel, what our goals are, and what our pain points or struggles are. These conversations can reveal that men have their own body insecurities too, and they can be a great place to solicit involvement in our body-positivity journey from the one we love most. It all starts with open communication.

I recently asked my husband what he thought the most attractive feature is in a woman. Without missing a beat, he gave his answer: confidence. And though I think it can be hard to believe that given how wrapped up we become in our own insecurities, I've leaned into that. The hardest part? Giving ourselves *permission* to be confident when the world tells us that our bodies are broken, bruised, flawed, or less than. Yet, as we know by now, there's only one person who can give us that permission: ourselves. We weren't created to be perfect—after all, we were sculpted from dust! We're bound to have some defects, but owning those and resting in the confidence that our bodies are sufficiently sexy as is can be wonderfully liberating.

Ultimately, love is a complicated game, and our complicated relationships with our bodies can make it even more difficult to navigate. But that difficulty comes from impositions *we* make. Whether you're currently with your forever Prince Charming or still searching for the one, the work you do to believe your body is good and to love it as it is, where it is, and how it is will only help you further ignite the fire in that relationship and in the sheets.

Flip the Script

Instead of telling yourself, "No one could ever love this body (naked)," say this instead: **"My body is beautiful, and I am worthy of being loved exactly as I am."**

Reflect

What hang-ups do you have about your body when it comes to sex and romance? How has your view of your body affected your relationships over the years? Or, if you've not found that special someone yet, how does your view of your body affect the way you feel about your intimate relationship with your future spouse?

Action Step

Next time you catch a glance of your naked self in the mirror, smile and say out loud, *"Gracious! You sure look good naked!"* Add a smile and a wink to drive the message home.

Chapter 5

FREE AND UNFILTERED

I've never been arrested, but I've lived in a prison my whole life. By now you know that the bars that have held me captive are not made of iron but of flesh and blood—the psychological barriers that held me down for far too long, keeping me from living freely and being fully me. I would argue that many of us find ourselves in this prison. We're used to seeing life through the filter of the bars in front of our faces.

But something occurs to me . . . this prison we find ourselves in—the one that has become a "normal" part of our lives—*this prison is not fatness.*

Let me say it louder for the people in the back. *This prison is not fatness.*

What holds us back is not our muffin tops, our cookie-dough arms, or even our drumstick legs. It's time we are honest with ourselves. I have had to step back and recognize that it wasn't my fat that held me back.

It was me.

And also, it was you. You held me back. I was striving for my full potential, and you knocked me off course.

I have been looking to you, watching you, studying you. You see your stretch marks; I see how many more I have. You see your double chin, but I can't get past the fact that I have a triple chin. For every negative you see in you, I see more in me.

The truth is that when your entire psyche has been wired to operate from a place of "I'm too fat" or "I'm too flawed," you can only find your identity by looking at the world around you to understand the space you inhabit. Through this flawed way of thinking, you can only understand *you* by seeing how you fit with—or stand in opposition to—*others*. I do not actually believe we compare ourselves out of a desperate desire to be as skinny or as muscular as someone else. We do it because we are so at odds with our own appearances, our own bodies, our own self-esteem, that we reach for anything and everything that will help reassure us that *we're not the worst*.

In order to ensure we're not at the absolute bottom of the totem pole, we fix our gaze on the people around us. We size them up one by one and align ourselves accordingly. We take a quick scroll through someone's Instagram profile. If she's leagues ahead of us, we want to be her. If she doesn't measure up, she's not worth our time.

Sometimes we're not quite that critical. We simply use the women around us as a safety net to ensure we're okay the way we are. And if we find we don't meet the standard, if most people seem above us in the pecking order, we work harder. We put more pressure on ourselves and hope that we'll one day get it right.

Then there are the times when we view the incredible people around us as a means of inspiration. If she can do it, so can I. But no matter the valence—positive or negative—we need to recognize three things:

- First, the culture of comparison is toxic, and it is destroying us from the inside out.
- Second, we have no one to blame but ourselves for further perpetuating it.
- Third, only we can break this cycle.

To talk about how we want it to end, we first have to think about where it begins.

PERFECT(LY ENHANCED) PHOTOS

Perhaps my only addiction worse than pizza is the one I (used to) have with social media. I'm young(ish), but I'm old enough to remember the days when you could toss on your prettiest dress, do your makeup real nice, curl your hair, and take a gander in the mirror to admire your work. That's where the process *ended*. Now it's just the beginning. I know I'm not the only woman who has all but scheduled time before my family leaves the house—for church, the mall, or a flight—to snap some images. I like to believe that this process was altruistic and that I was simply trying to document the fleeting moments with my children and my husband. But I know this isn't entirely true. I did it as a reflection of who I was.

Now I'm going to give us all some grace here. We aren't so egocentric that we're posting photos only for likes or comments. We've simply been hardwired to see this as normal. Selfie culture has bled into our day-to-day life so strongly that now many of us can only see ourselves through filters. Our lives aren't about the events we attend; they're centered completely upon how we've documented those events.

In and of itself, snapping life's moments in our digital memory Rolodex is not harmful or toxic. But so many dimensions to this process should cause us to step back and question whether it is as innocent as it seems. Pastor Holly Furtick once commented in a sermon just how ironic it is that our social media spaces are called *feeds*. We go there when we're hungry—not physically, but emotionally—and we fill our minds with food for thought for later.[1]

I'd never look as good as she does in a scoop neck.

She's always so happy. She must not have the same struggles as the rest of us.

She's the perfect mom with the perfect body—how does that even happen?

So, we respond with posts of our own. And we don't just snap a photo—we take a hundred photos and choose the one where our muffin top is contained, our chin is appropriately positioned, and our wrinkles are concealed. We don't just upload a photo to Instagram—we edit it, apply a filter, and try to hide the things we don't like about ourselves. We smooth and brighten our skin, suck in our guts, remove blemishes, and crop out the part that makes our arms look wider than we like. All because we need every single photo to appear "just right."

The problem is that the appropriately positioned "just right" me doesn't really exist. What you see in someone's Instagram photo looks perfect, but the truth of the matter is that it is just *perfectly enhanced.* We can make ourselves look better in thirty seconds or less. Some of us are good at it, some not so much. I see photos all the time where I have to step back and say, "Whoa—that is not who I thought it was" because the alterations were so significant.

And honestly, we do this because it works. That effort comes with a reward. The comments, likes, and shout-outs we get on social media give our brains a huge dose of feel-good brain juice. We thrive on this feedback, and instead of seeing it for what it is, we reframe it under the lens of positivity—*hooray for women empowering one another!* We do need to empower one another, and in fact I would argue that we need to be more liberal in dishing out kind comments to each other. Social media is a hard place to be a woman. But when I compliment a sister, I want her to know that I'm complimenting the *real* her—what she brings to the table in her skills, her talents, her passion, her creativity, her energy. I'm not doing her any good by flattering a well-choreographed and digitized caricature of who she is.

Over dinner a few weeks ago, I got to chatting with a fellow "momtrepreneur" whose children are a few years older than mine. Her daughter had been online, scrolling through ideas for her upcoming birthday party. She wanted an over-the-top, magical celebration with all the works. When she found photos of an idea that looked amazing, she kept begging her mom to make it happen for her, pleading that this would be the defining moment of her adolescent life. Like all moms (me included), my friend felt pressure to make her daughter's day as special and exciting as possible. But this mom said something to her daughter that struck me so deeply. In her gentle way, she helped her daughter understand that no matter how amazing the party was, it would never feel quite as perfect and amazing as the pictures she'd found made it seem.

That's a huge lesson for a nine-year-old but an even greater one for us grown-ups. We see perfection everywhere we look but fail to realize that it's often staged. We're so focused on achieving perfection that we don't realize it's entirely fabricated. Lost in the pursuit of perfection, we fail to step back and live in our own moments—moments filled with

> We see perfection everywhere we look but fail to realize that it's often staged.

imperfection, mishaps, messy hair, and actual connection with other *real* people and the *real* world around us.

This is a good moment for a balance check. Yes, we need to be real, but that doesn't mean we can't change our reality. I mean, the *real* you in the morning has breath that smells like death and the grave. That isn't the *real* you that I particularly want to encounter until you brush those teeth and scrub your tongue. I'm not saying that you're wrong—that *we're* wrong—for making changes. I'm all for chopping off your hair and trying a pixie cut, or a crazy color, or Botox, or breast reconstruction. Making changes to your body is not innately declaring that you hate your body. Bodies are not robots created on an assembly line; they are meant to be personalized as an extension of the creativity that God gave us. No two are exactly alike.

I've changed my body composition countless times. From gaining, to losing, to gaining again, to losing again, to working on muscle build, to carrying babies, to losing weight again, to getting skin surgery, to finding a good skin care line to clarify my sun spots, to drastically changing my hair color several times, to . . .

Change is *good*, and it keeps things fresh and exciting.

But this is where we come back to motive. What drives the changes? Are they coming from a place of deep dissatisfaction or a healthy place of contentment? Are you making changes to get a response from people, or are you doing it for yourself? We need to dig deeper and ensure that we're not addicted to the affirmations of others. If we're making changes—whether in person or through Photoshop—in a desperate attempt to one day reach an impossible standard of beauty, we'll be reaching forever and we'll never be satisfied.

YOUR BODY, MY BODY, EVERYBODY

It's amazing how fast someone else's social media post can derail our positivity. I can look at a photo of myself and think I'm sure lookin' cute, but ten seconds later when I scroll, feeding my mind with the perfection feed, I often feel like all of that means nothing because *she* always. looks. so. good. Even when I fully (re)commit myself to the most mindful pursuit of health and wellness, I am amazed at how I am sidetracked by *her*, who dropped ten pounds without trying. Or *her*, who used to share a pear shape with me but doesn't any longer. What is she doing? Can I do that? Am I way off in my pursuit? Why isn't it working for me? As much as I want to celebrate another woman's meaningful progress alongside her, I have to remember that *her* progress doesn't mean my failure. The steps forward she's making in her journey don't mean steps lost in mine.

The comparison trap rears its ugly head on all levels and in so many different ways. In fact, entire works have been written on this concept alone. But this book isn't just about comparison; it's about comparison within a specific domain—our bodies.

I've often wondered what the final answer is to how big I am. Am I still considered fat at the size I am today? Some people tell me I look small, but I think that's just because they've seen me at my biggest. Quite honestly, I've spent more time confused about my own size than I'd like to admit. For a while, I was embarrassed to offer fitness tips and share about healthy living because I was pretty sure people thought, *Well, who is she to talk?* At the same time, I was scared to talk about body positivity because I knew some people didn't actually see me the way *I* see me, so they didn't understand why I had negative thought patterns I needed to change.

Am I fat? Skinny? Medium? Built? Curvy? Fluffy? It all depends on who you ask. If you ask me, you're likely to receive any range of answers depending on the day or hour or minute—and who I'm comparing myself to at that moment. If I'm comparing myself to 336-pound Jennifer, well then, I'd probably say I fall on the smaller side. If I'm comparing myself to those fitness gurus at the gym who have become some of my best friends, well then, I'd probably say I'm chunky. Strong! But chunky.

That can be a hard identity battle to fight—to be double-minded in your ways, thinking that you're small in one context, big in another. You start to fall prey again to the idea that your health can only be understood by your size and the space you occupy. And then you find yourself in an unhealthy place where the comparison trap has overwritten your true underlying goals and motivations. It took me 50,000 times of walking around this circle to realize that it honestly doesn't matter how others see me. The only thing that matters is how

I see myself; I am only productive when I refuse to compare myself to anyone else.

We see that all bodies are different, but even in the midst of a "health at every size" wave of acceptance, we still find it difficult to embrace the idea that bodies are—or should be—*truly different.* If we really bought into the idea that bodies are good at every size and shape, we would abandon the cycle of self-loathing that defines so much of our lives.

Comparing our bodies to someone else's never brings anything good. We have it all wrong where this is concerned. We think that hating ourselves into submission is going to work. We assume that change happens the way it did when we were kids: We're "bad," then we get "corrected" through harsh words or reprimands, and then we become "good." We apply the same process when it comes to trying to change our bodies. We're so punitive when it comes to our "bad" eating or "lazy" exercise habits. We suspect that if we punish ourselves for desiring decadence and taking pleasure in excess, or if we reprimand ourselves enough for not looking as good as the next person on our feed, for not pushing hard enough, or for not succeeding, eventually everything will fall into place.

It won't.

I can tell you from firsthand experience that if you are striving to "get healthy" to scratch an itch created by another person, later on you'll find a whole new set of issues to work through. The truth is, there will always be someone to compare yourself to, fostering yet another itch to scratch. No matter what level you achieve—in life, in your health, in your fitness, in your journey—you will *always* find someone who is just that much further ahead of you in the game. You'll work harder and harder, and though it might feel empowering for a while, eventually your physical being and your emotional being will meet up for coffee and realize they're incompatible. And when those two are out of sync, it quickly leads to burnout.

We can wrap our heads around this principle more easily in a different context. Think of it like an appetite for money. If you know people who are actively chasing money, I'm betting they can't rest because they are always in pursuit of more. A new car isn't enough—they need a better model as soon as they see their neighbor with one. One luxury handbag isn't enough—they have to have a step up from what their coworkers carry. There's nothing wrong with having or spending money. But when money is all you think about, it consumes you in a way that renders the rest of your life largely useless. The same is true for health and fitness. There's nothing wrong with it; in fact, it's good for you. But if you see it as the be-all and end-all of your life, if you spend all your time comparing your results with others', you will falter in your efforts. Not to mention, you'll miss out on a whole lot of life you could have experienced if you'd loosened your grip ever so slightly.

FREE TO BE ME 3-D

Our culture of comparison thrives predominantly because it is so one-note. It's easy to compare ourselves to others because we aren't really comparing ourselves to others—we're comparing one-dimensional, point-in-time artifacts to each other. We're comparing apples to apples—photo to photo, if you will. But when we bring those one-dimensional accounts of our lives to life, we recognize that we aren't comparing apples to apples anymore. It's apples and oranges. Apples and tuna salad. Apples and giraffes.

The inner workings of our design are individual. We were created with an individual purpose and set apart to walk on a dynamic path that was prepared just for us. Beyond the surface level, every one of us contains layer upon layer of experiences that have made us who we are today. Yet because we're running full-speed ahead, we naturally boil down all processes—even human interaction—to their most simple element. As we orient ourselves in the greater human land-scape, we do so by comparing the one-dimensional "image" we present of ourselves to others' one-dimensional images. We're so overburdened with information that this becomes the easiest way to understand who we are and how we fit in the world around us.

But people have so much more depth than we naturally perceive. We reduce people to the fifteen seconds it took for them to snap a perfect image and forget about the other 86,385 seconds that make up their days. What we deem as truth and fact is merely a fractional account of the much bigger picture.

When I finally realized that I was in a constant state of anxiety about my body, even *after* losing a massive amount of weight, it wasn't long before I figured out that people don't actually care about my body as much as I think they do. Sure, my peers during my childhood and teen years cared—but maybe only because they were looking for an easy target for jokes and teasing. Most adults have moved past that stage. And so, while I was preoccupied with the way my legs rubbed together when I walked into a room, the rest of the world hadn't thought a thing of it. The reward I got for not showing off my flabby arms in a T-shirt, choosing to slip into something a bit more "upper arm modest" instead? Not a darn thing. The truth of the matter is that the people I interact with on an interpersonal level are generally not evaluating my body at all. And, fun fact, if they are, they're usually doing it because of a major insecurity of their own. (See? It all comes full circle.)

What I've discovered is that people want the real me. They want to hear the struggle; they want to *see* the struggle. I'd be a liar if I said that I'm ready to bare it all to the world. But if you scroll through my own social media feed, you'll also see that I try to show more of "me"—not just the good, but the ugly too. Not just the perfectly positioned, but also the natural.

I finally pushed back on my tendency to post only showstoppers when my husband snapped a (ridiculously cute) photo of my toddler son playing with my belly fat. Apparently, the squishiness of my fluff was more fun than his toys, and I was perfectly happy letting him grab it by the handful. Never wanting my kids to see fat in a negative context, I'm not offended by them noticing the bigness of my legs or, in this case, the moldable texture of my tummy. In fact, this happened at a time when I'd really started thinking about this whole body-positivity thing. I'd already lost all the weight I was going to lose (and put about fifteen pounds back on), and I was tired of having a thousand reasons to hate my body.

So, I embraced it. And I posted the photo. No retouching, or airbrushing, or filters. I wanted people to see what I saw when I looked at my son's face that day. There wasn't an ounce of disgust in his eyes. No judgment or disappointment. The only thing on his mind was that whatever this stuff in his hands was, it was fun to play with. And since Mommy didn't seem to mind, it must not be such a bad thing.

I'd never posted anything like that before, and I pushed the share button with unexpected butterflies. The real, raw Jennifer—that's what the social media world was getting that day. I don't know how I expected everyone to respond, but for as long as it took to post it, I didn't care. I so desperately wanted to see the reality of my own body without shuddering in angst. At the same time, I wanted other women—women just like me and totally different from me—to see that our bodies are good. Just as they are.

Since then, I've gotten more intentional about being less careful in what I post. I have found that I have so much more to offer those around me, and this can be best accomplished when I'm not caught up in some pursuit of ever-fleeting perfection. I'm not only helping me, I'm helping those I encounter both on social media and in real life. I'm reminded that when I've been with others in person and they leave my presence, their thoughts are not filled with a checklist of the ways in which my body did or did not align to some pseudo standard that I might be obsessed with. They are going to remember the words I spoke to them. The authenticity of my demeanor, my attentiveness when they spoke. The kindness that I extended toward them, the warmth of my hug. The consistency of my friendship. They're going to remember *how I made them feel.*

The difference between a one-dimensional life and a three-dimensional life comes down to this: the power of feeling authentically connected and valued. The images of perfection that we present and consume make us feel "less than" because those posts often come from a place of self-doubt and anxiety. When we live three-dimensionally, though, our caricature of perfection rises above a mere digital image and comes to life. By living life out loud—flaws and all—we can help others feel better about themselves, recognizing that they don't have to have it all together. And perhaps even more importantly, we can help ourselves feel better. When we're willing to show our imperfections, we're telling the comparison trap that it's far too inhibiting for us. We see our value, and we know that it goes beyond how our chins, arms, and bellies look. Our value lies in the power we have to impact and drive positive change in the world around us.

One-dimensional me knows how to look pretty, but

three-dimensional me can show you that there's much more to me than meets the eye. There's a whole person beyond what you see on the surface. I have feelings, talents, abilities, dreams, and gifts to offer to the world around me. And so do you.

This is where true freedom lies. Freedom comes when we understand that our worth is not determined by the attributes of our bodies. The depths of who we are are manifested in living, breathing humans that are much more than just the sum of our physical attributes. Freedom comes when we focus more on who we are as collective beings than on our curves and fluff.

> Freedom comes when we understand that our worth is not determined by the attributes of our bodies.

Overwhelming freedom comes when we learn to love our bodies completely as they are today, without the guarantee of a refund when we notice something we deem as less than the standard of perfection. *Ultimate* freedom comes when we abandon the idea of perfection altogether.

You are so much more than meets the eye. Who you are as a three-dimensional person means more to me than that one-dimensional account of what you would like to be. When we make the decision to love ourselves as we are and pursue health in a balanced way, we will begin looking to ourselves instead of social media to discover who we are and what we're worth. We'll start to find peace, stability, and comfort by looking within instead of comparing ourselves to others around us.

- Your kids love you for your awesome mom skills—not your six-pack.
- Your husband loves you no matter if you have one love handle or two. And he loves *you*—not just your body.
- Your friends appreciate your quirks and value your companionship and could care less about the size or shape of your thighs.
- Your boss thinks you're a rock star, not because of how you fill out a business-casual dress but because of the value you bring to your work environment.
- I think you're amazing because you're taking the time to read, study, and improve your life on your own terms. I don't care if you're 90 pounds or 390 pounds.

You are not a simplistic reduction. You're so much more. Don't do yourself a disservice by falling prey to the comparison trap. Comparison robs you of joy. It fills your heart with negativity about yourself and makes you feel inadequate. Comparison also robs you of time. Hours upon hours spent subconsciously pondering the lived experience of everyone else leaves you empty on time you could have spent focusing on enjoying the world around you. And comparison robs you of quality of life. Instead of obsessing about what could be or what you wish your body was like, focus on the here and now. Spend the same energy you invest on anxiety in enjoying where life has you at this moment.

Reframe comparison with a radically simple declaration

that the only person you'll compare yourself to is *you*. Compare your today to yesterday and do what you can to make it count even more. Compare *this* body to the body of yesteryear (even if it's bigger, flabbier, more saggy, or more wrinkly). Remember what *this* body has carried you through. Thank this body. Compare your old way of thinking to a new one—a way of thinking that subscribes to the idea that you are good just the way you are.

Flip the Script

Instead of telling yourself, "I hate how I look in photos," say this instead: **"One picture is a millisecond snapshot, and I'm a whole entire human."**

Reflect

What role does comparison play in your life? How has comparison negatively affected your view of yourself?

Action Step

Post an unfiltered photo that communicates something about who you are beyond your appearance. Unfollow people who make you feel bad about yourself. This is *your* journey.

Chapter 6

BREAKING UP WITH THE SCALE

Perhaps it's the mama bear in me, but when my hubby's out of town, I walk through my house thinking about the items that I could use to create a makeshift weapon if someone broke in. Just in case. I like to think I'd be able to Jodie Foster an intruder right out of my house with my Ikea rolling pin, but if not, at least I have a mental inventory of items that can save the day if necessary.

If needed, I can grab the vacuum cleaner, a dresser drawer, or maybe even a chair from the dining room table.

But recently, as I was doing my (yes, I know it's absolutely ridiculous) inventory of items that would pack a punch, I came across a weapon lying on my bathroom floor.

Suddenly it dawned on me that this thing packs the biggest punch of all.

It was the scale. Only I wasn't thinking about how I could knock out a burglar by throwing it at him. No, I was struck by the thought of how much damage that thing used to inflict on *me* every single day. You'd think that the author of a book on how to love your body would have some magic formula for grappling with the scale. And while I'd like to tell you that the scale and I have been good friends forever, the truth of the matter is that our relationship took years of effort to become what it is. For years we were decidedly *not good*. Superman has his kryptonite, and I have mine (though mine is a lot less interesting to fight on the big screen).

Weight is a unit of measurement. In its simplest form, weight tells us a tale of the impact gravity has on our human bodies. But often, the scale's stories are instead accounts of anxiety. Dread. Denial. And, in what's a central concept for this book, worth.

WEIGHT AND WORTH

We frequently put weight and worth together. We often think in economic terms—for example, weighing the pros and cons of something by calculating how much value it adds. We weigh an apple in the grocery store so we know how much it will cost. We weigh the options when buying a new purse or car. We weigh our babies regularly to make sure they are growing and successfully moving toward adulthood. In most of our encounters, weight and value go hand in hand.

However, when it comes to our physical bodies, instead of seeing the value as a mere number, we've internalized what the scale tells us to be an indication of our actual value in the world around us. We've distorted the idea of value. In fact, conversations about our physical weight are the only context that I can think of where *less* means *more* and *more* means *less*. In this chapter I want to pull back our expectations of the scale and, particularly, what it means about our worth.

I am not against using a scale. I believe in health and wellness (which sometimes intersects with weight gain or loss but is never exclusively body-size driven), but I do not believe the scale tells us everything we need to know. I'm not saying you should never use a scale again. I get it; seeking health without some sort of check-and-balance system is a tricky ask. But what if we could see the scale for what it is (a tool for measurement) and stop seeing it for what it isn't (a measure of our worth)?

Let's talk about that stupid scale.

IT REALLY IS STUPID

I don't let my kids say the word *stupid* for the same reason I don't let them say other strong words. But if I'm going to cut to the chase here, I have to admit that the scale is pretty . . . stupid.

The basic definition of stupidity is lacking intelligence

or knowledge. The scale has neither. It's a flat piece of metal or plastic with some batteries thrown in. It has no intellect. It cannot breathe, eat, walk, or solve even the simplest math problem. It can do nothing—except spew technologically calculated numbers at us.

And that it does. Its language is simple and universal—it just spits out what gravity tells it to.

336.

299.

261.

204.

227.

187.

124.

144.

166.

179.

185.

The scale is perfectly content to spurt out a response to the question that many of us ask it: *What am I worth today?* It has answered me every time I've asked. Some days, the scale is quite the flatterer; other days, it's quite a jerk. But on all days, the scale is right there waiting for me. Like a big, ugly meanie . . . that I keep coming back to time and time again.

WHY WE HATE THE SCALE

There are many reasons why we hate the scale, and they range from one to whatever number you see when you stand on it. But I think this is far too simple. By blaming the stupid scale for the lack of progress we want to see, we take the easy way out. We make numbers the enemy when numbers are only a tool.

Numbers have value, but they have no meaning until we *give* it to them. The same is true with money. All US dollars look essentially the same. They are green, rectangular, and covered in germs. In the middle there's a dead president or statesman, whose image corresponds to a specific number. If you closed your eyes, you'd have no idea how much the cash in your wallet was worth. But each bill holds its value based on how it's designated.

It's similar for weight. We can see the number, but until we have a collective understanding of what that number means, it's a meaningless statistic that has no inherent value. We have to understand that while that number can help us calibrate where we stand and where we're heading, it can't tell us everything about who we are or even how healthy we are. It simply does not paint the full picture.

We've got to get over our obsession with the scale. I talk to a lot of women all across the country and even across the globe about health and wellness. Inevitably, very early on in every conversation, the scale comes into the picture. After so many conversations, I've been able to synthesize what I believe are the key reasons people hate the scale. They all come down to the way they've *personalized* it. We've let the scale take on an identity.

The IRS

I love four out of the five seasons. Spring, summer, autumn, and winter are all fine by me. But April 15 has to be my least favorite holiday, even though it ends the most dreaded season of all: tax season. In the United States, we're fortunate enough to pay taxes to the tune of about 30 percent of our income. That's huge when you think about it. But we know that taxes serve a good purpose. They help provide for our roads and infrastructures, they keep us safe and protected, and they fund many programs that help our country function. Still—it isn't fun to have to pay those taxes.

I can't help but see the scale as yet another arm of the IRS, there to collect something from me. Often, I feel like I owe it—like I have to pay a price just for living. Maybe I'm alone here, but when I've looked down at the number the scale spits out, I've literally said, "I'm sorry" out loud when I've come up short (or, actually, just the opposite). Other times, I've gotten so mad at the scale because I felt like *it owed me*. (I won't type out the things I've said to it in case there are kids in the room. Kidding. Sort of.) Know how when you overpay the IRS, you get that glorious tax-return check back in the mail? So many times I've stepped on that square piece of metal expecting to see the fruits of my hard labor throughout the previous week, only to be robbed of what I felt was owed me.

I have to remind myself that the scale doesn't have the intellectual capacity to sense my efforts and take them into account when it calculates its output. I owe the scale nothing and, though it's an even harder truth to grapple with, the scale owes me nothing. This is not a financial interaction.

The Boss

I've had a lot of good bosses over the years. In fact, I've been privileged to develop a close relationship with almost all of them. But I distinctly remember one boss, in my early years, who was awful to work for. Her micromanaging tendencies were the absolute worst. In my youthful desire to do a great job in the workplace, I began to make myself crazy trying to live up to the wildly detailed expectations of an employer who could never be fully pleased or proud of a job well done.

She said jump, and I asked how high. There was no need to develop a good working relationship or rapport; it was boss and subordinate. Period.

I think the same thing can be true for our relationship with the scale. We see it as *the boss.* The tough talker. The one who knows how to call the shots. A boss is often one who sits on high monitoring our progress, ensuring that our input (work) is worth his or her output (money). We've come to treat the scale as the ultimate boss. We clock in every day when we step on it and then we go about performing the "work" we need to do in order to appease the scale and get its approval. We're always hoping that our paycheck (the scale's output) will reflect and honor that hard work.

But again, we've given the scale too much power. Take the batteries out and what good is it? It's not a good boss. Good bosses pour into you and care about your development. They know who you are and what makes you qualified to fit in their company. But the scale? It can't do that! It doesn't care! It has nothing substantial to offer because it has no invest-ment in us. It only displays what it calculates. Here's the truth of the matter: Bosses who *tell it like it is* are never great bosses anyway. *Good* bosses are collaborators. They come alongside you, using their talents to help you cultivate yours, and as a result, you flourish.

To some extent, the scale is capable of holding that same partnership with us. Its numbers can help us calibrate where we are as we journey toward our healthiest selves. But it's not in charge; we are. So if you're seeing it as a boss, take it down a few pegs and make sure you're seeing it as one of many tools of measurement, not the dictator of your health or assessor of your value as a person.

The Parent

You can't exactly fire your parents. Though believe me, as a teenager, I did look into it. I'll readily admit that I wasn't the easiest person to raise. I had a good heart, but yikes—those teenage years were tough! I'm surprised my mom didn't lose her mind trying to pull through that awful stint of prepubes-cent hormones and roller-coaster emotions.

Nothing has made me appreciate and empathize with all the mommies of the world like having my own children. There are so many things I do every single day that I swore I would *never* do as a parent. I thought I had parenthood completely figured out, but then I became a mom and realized that all my presuppositions went right out the window along with every ounce of confidence in my ability to do the job on the most challenging days.

No one exactly teaches you how to be a good parent. People teach you how to get pregnant (the fun part) and how to give birth (arguably not as fun), but no one prepares you for the real shock of actual parenthood. Through all the highs it brings, I think we can admit that it's quite difficult. Why? Because parenting has so many unforeseen *not fun* parts. In our pursuit to raise kind, loving, respectful, contributing members of society who actually function and operate as wholesome, healthy human beings, we have a lot of "no" moments.

Mom, can I have another cookie? No.

Mom, can you wipe my butt? No—you're five. Figure it out, honey.

Mom, can I jump off the roof into the swimming pool? No, baby. Just . . . no.

As lovely as my parents were, I remember feeling like every answer they gave was a hard and fast no. "You *always* say no!" I'd yell at the top of my lungs when I didn't get my way.

And now as I sit here writing these words, I'm realizing we regard the scale the same way. We see it as something there to ensure we have no fun at all.

No good food.

No days off.

Just lots of work, deprivation, and temptations I can't give into.

If we let it, the scale will be a decent parent. Not a good one—not the kind that puts a Band-Aid on your wounds or tucks you in at night—but one that will keep you accountable and "safe." But for most of us, seeing the scale as a parent evokes a reaction similar to an earth-shattering teenage outburst. We rebel against even well-intended guidelines because we don't want to be under someone else's control or authority. When we quit thinking of the scale as a parent and more as a tool, we take more responsibility for ourselves. We feel like we're in charge. We make the choices not because we're afraid of discipline or correction, but because we've matured to the point of trusting the growth process.

The Doctor

No one *likes* to go to the doctor. Blood. Needles. Gauze.

The scale.

What is with that old-timey scale they use? After all, we're well into the twenty-first century. *Can't y'all get some modern scales?* But no—whether it be out of some medical necessity or for the sake of a good old nostalgic dramatic effect, those nurses love to slide their fingers over the heavy clinkers of that archaic weighing device. Often I pity them. Either they go way overboard and have to backtrack (how offensive), or they go way under and then have to flick it up a few dozen pounds (how depressing). For much of my life, I hated the scale so much that I just looked the other direction as they tinkered around to find their precise measurement of my body. Yes, I was that committed to protesting the scale.

I've even had a conversation about this with my doctors, who are all ever-patient with my constant anxieties about health. We had a serious conversation several years ago about my unhealthy fixation with the scale. I was *so* focused on the number. I just couldn't understand why I, a person whose entire life existence was wrapped up in this identity of a weight-loss aficionado, still saw the number that I saw on the scale. I was convinced that meant something was wrong. I asked about everything you could imagine:

"It's my thyroid, isn't it? It has to be."

"Ah, I'm probably pregnant. Please tell me I'm pregnant. But please don't make me tell my husband I'm pregnant."

"Oh wow . . . I must be holding water. Do you think it's because I shower three times a day? Should I back off? Maybe too much salt?"

"Cancer. Oh my gosh. It's cancer, isn't it? That's clearly the only reason I weigh this much. How big is the tumor?"

My doctor finally sat down, looked me in the eye, and had an honest conversation with me:

"The scale is not the doctor. I am. I know you want it to say a certain number but, honey, you're healthier than 95 percent of the people who come in here. Every single test I ran for you came back absolutely

> The scale doesn't have a medical degree. It is certainly not qualified to diagnose me. So why am I giving it power?

fantastic. Your resting heart rate is that of an athlete. Good grief, you're healthier than me!"

And in that moment, it finally sank in. The scale doesn't have a medical degree. The stupid thing has never gotten a formal education of any kind. It is certainly not qualified to diagnose me. So why am I giving it power? The scale is a tool, but it is not a diagnostic; it cannot tell you about your entire health journey. Let's make sure we aren't conferring upon it a medical degree it didn't earn.

The Other Woman

As you know by reading the other chapters, my husband is a certified saint. He loved me when I was at my biggest and often fails to see my size altogether. The dude loves me for who I am, where I am—period. Yet no matter how many times he's told me this and no matter how many times I've told him that I understand, we often keep coming back to a defining fight in our marriage: the one about *the other woman.*

Relax, he didn't cheat on me. He isn't my problem; I'm my own problem. I've invited the scale to define so much of my identity. Try as I might, I have a hard time shaking the feminine expectations that our image-consumed world has of women like me. We're expected to be fit and mindful of our size but never so much that we outpace the men in our lives. Perfectly chiseled in the gym, but not at the consequence of neglecting our children or household duties. It's no wonder then that we all seek some fictionalized version of ourselves—the "other woman" who acts like us, sounds like us, talks like us, and thinks like us—but is *just so much more perfect.* The scale can become the symbol of this for us; we think if we just reached our goal weight, we could stop envying that other woman and actually become her.

But here's the thing: By constantly seeking fictionalized versions of ourselves, we're neglecting the value of who we are, right here and right now. As such, we're missing out on the precious moments that we could spend on cultivating relational depth and satisfaction.

A friend of mine who used to be quite thin (her description, not mine) once confided her frustrations about how her body has changed over the years. As time and gravity have taken their tolls, her body changed quite significantly, as all of ours do. She wants to enjoy the beautiful season of life she's in now, but sometimes she mourns the loss of what she once had—a youthful body with a smaller dress size.

She's constantly wrestling with another woman: her former self. But at her core she's the same self she was back then. Only now she's been polished with life experiences: her kids' birthday parties, pizza nights, career demands, highs, lows, you name it. Her body has carried babies, raised them, and kept up with caring for their every need. She's grown in wisdom. She's developed in love. Her heart is filled with compassion more than ever before. She seeks to live up to the physique of that younger woman who taunts her but forgets that she is, in fact, that same woman, only a beautifully flourishing and seasoned version.

It's not the weight or size of your body that makes you the incredible woman you are, nor would you be more worthy if you did finally attain that body composition you reminisce about. You are enough, my friend. As you are today. Maybe you've been thinner; maybe you're the fittest you've ever been. Maybe health is your permanent lifestyle and maybe you're just testing the waters. No matter what, I want to encourage you to stop seeking *the other woman* and start developing the healthiest version of who *you* are today. You are not the old you and, blunt truth, you are not the future you. Both are optimistic versions of you that you're likely viewing through rose-colored glasses.

Don't let the scale drive your pursuit of a different you or even hearken you back to yesteryear. Don't give it that power. You don't need to search for another woman; you're enough. Don't let the scale tell you otherwise.

TRY THIS, NOT THAT

If we refuse to let the scale play all of these roles in our lives, it loses its power. It becomes a neutral tool that you can use if you want to. Truth be told, I use the scale from time to time. But the beauty in where I am now is that regardless of what the scale says, I don't fall apart. I never thought I'd be able to use the scale as a means of helping me navigate my habits without linking it to my mood for the entire day. But here

I am. My only wish is that I could have come to a healthier relationship with the scale a very long time ago.

So what do you do, then, if you must face this behemoth of a villain? How do you face the monster that causes you so much anxiety and invite it to go along with you on your journey to health? I've found that it takes soul-searching. We have to ensure first and foremost that we are ready to face whatever reality the scale gives us with an understanding that it's just one small part of our overall health journey. I've also found that checking our assumptions about what "number" equals health can go a long way. When you stand on that 12 x 12 black box, don't let it tell you what you're worth; tell *it* what you're worth and celebrate what the numbers say because they show that you're a human. You get to define your worth, not the scale.

At this point in my journey, I weigh myself whenever I feel like it. Sometimes it's more frequent, other times I don't bother with it for a while. But what's made a huge difference to me is that after I strip off all my clothes, I pause. I look in the mirror and appreciate my body for a second. Then, when my mind is ready, I step on the scale and use the number as a gauge. That moment of appreciation—of seeing my body as good—has alleviated so much of my scale anxiety.

We can *use* the scale as long as we do not allow it to tell us a tale about our value. Or we can break up with it and throw it in the garbage can.

If you aren't ready for the big breakup just yet, I would

like to offer you some mindset shifts that can begin to free you from the angst that often comes with the scale. Maybe when you're ready you'll sever the ties, but until then, here are some things to consider:

If your weight is higher than it was last time, consider some of the common reasons why that might happen:

- The scale can reflect some really hard work. After a particularly intense workout, muscles can expand and fill with water. If that's the case, it means you're getting stronger. Time to celebrate!
- The scale can tell you about what is happening in your body. Are you on your menstrual cycle? Could there be something happening within you that is causing your body to hold on to weight? Give grace and time for your body to do what it needs to.
- Could you be holding water? Traveling, eating out, or consuming more salt than usual can all cause temporary water retention, which is absolutely normal.
- Have you restricted your calorie consumption? Is your body fighting a war inside of you, holding on to any stored fat you have because you're being a stubborn mule and refusing to eat? Your body needs food, my friend.

If your weight is the same as last time, here is what the scale is not *saying*:

- It is *not* saying you failed. You didn't.
- It is *not* saying you didn't work hard enough. You did.
- It is *not* saying that you did something wrong. There is no "right" or "wrong" here—these are just numbers.
- It is *not* saying that terrible thing you always think about yourself. You're saying that. Shift your thinking.

If your weight is lower than last time, remember to spot-check your emotions:

- Losing weight doesn't make your body good or bad.
- Losing weight doesn't make you better today than the *you* of yesterday.
- Losing weight doesn't change your worth.
- Losing weight doesn't change who you are.
- Losing weight doesn't lead to automatic happiness.
- Losing weight isn't permanent; remember that your body can (and should) change with the seasons of life. Whether that means a gain or a loss the next time you're on the scale, don't get so focused on the scale that it causes you to miss out on enjoying the ups and downs— the natural cadence—of life.

I'D BE HAPPY IF I WEIGHED . . .

What if your "happy weight"—the point where you can finally become content—has nothing to do with the actual number on a scale? As you begin to travel the road to freedom in your health journey, my hope is that you'll have a different barometer for what you're working toward. As we've discussed in this chapter, the number on a scale has very little bearing on how you feel and your overall health. In the next chapters, we'll talk about nourishing and moving our bodies in ways that contribute to our feeling energized, confident, and whole. We want to see progress in our health journeys, but can we set goals for ourselves that are more about how we feel, both physically

> We can pursue creative goals and track our progress without being chained to the scale.

and emotionally, and less about how we look or what we weigh? Maybe it's about seeking better overall health, increased energy or flexibility, lower blood pressure, or more confidence. We can pursue creative goals like this and track our progress without being chained to the scale.

What would happen if you thought outside the box for a moment and considered what you want life to look like at your "goal weight"? Because the truth of the matter is that your happiness may have nothing to do with that weight. What if your "goal weight" wasn't actually a *weight*, but rather a state of being free from scale anxiety, diet culture, and self-loathing? For so long we've thought the goal was to reach a BMI posted on the wall in the doctor's office, but I suspect that what we really want is to be free from feeling as though we are on a tightrope, tiptoeing through every bite of food we put into our mouths because we're afraid of gaining pounds.

I'm not telling you to throw your scale out the window, just as I am not telling you to weigh yourself twice a day. I can't tell you the absolute correct approach to when or how often to pull out the scale because that varies based on who you ask.

But what I can tell you is that adjusting your *relationship* with the scale can be life-changing. Maybe you're at the point right now where weighing yourself only brings you feelings of defeat or stress. If that's the case, feel free to take a good, long stretch of time (determined by you) away from the dang thing. Maybe you're at a place where you're fine with weighing yourself, and it's not bringing you anguish but instead a stress-free accountability. It is 100 percent your choice as to how you utilize the scale.

My current relationship with the scale did not happen overnight. I've gone through so many different approaches based on what I needed at the time. I've broken up with the scale before, I've weighed myself obsessively (not recommended!), I've lived in absolute fear of stepping on that thing (also not recommended!), you name it. But the best place I can be is one where I detach my value, and even my overall health, from that final number that pops on the screen when I stand on the scale.

The scale is a monster to be grappled with. At its worst, it is an unrestrained weapon of mass destruction. I know it has been for me. Now that I can easily hop on and off the scale without anxiety, I regret all the lies I used to believe.

Like thinking I could be reduced to a number. I can't.

Like thinking that the totality of my health journey can be tallied in pounds and ounces. It can't.

Like thinking that my body and its abilities are only measurable in ups and downs. They aren't.

I refuse to buy into these lies, and I refuse to be the same type of bully that the scale is. It isn't stupid—it just *is*. It is an inanimate object designed to meet a specific purpose. Let's make sure we have clear and justifiable expectations of the scale and don't give it more power than it's meant to hold.

Flip the Script

Instead of telling yourself, "I've got to drop at least ten pounds," say this instead: **"The scale does not determine my health or worth."**

Reflect

How do you view the scale? How might your "happy weight" actually be quite different from the number you had in mind as a "goal weight"?

Action Step

Write down your goal weight on a piece of paper—and then rip the paper into shreds and throw it in the trash. Next, write down how you'd like to feel physically and emotionally and use that as your goal instead of the number on the scale.

Chapter 7

MOVE YOUR GOOD BODY

The irony of my three-year-old screaming, "I'm tired! I don't wanna go!" in the back seat on our way to the gym wasn't lost on me that morning a few years ago. Cutting through the shrill sounds of his desperate pleas to ditch the gym in favor of watching yet another episode of something that is *totally educational* were my own internal toddler-esque tantrums. *I don't want to go either, buddy.*

This hasn't always been true, but in so many ways, the gym is my happy place. When COVID-19 hit and forced us all out of the gym and into our living rooms, I had a semi-meltdown. After all, the gym is the place where I rise from the ashes of my past and use movement—intense, deliberate, and forceful—to reclaim parts of my story. For those people who cut me down because of my size, I jog a little faster, lunge a little deeper, and sweat a little harder. And I haven't forgotten where I started. There was a time when I could barely walk a mile, and now I can crush an intense workout that would leave even some athletes passed out in a pool of sweat on the gym floor.

But also . . . I'm human and kind of hate it sometimes too. My muscles scream at me when I'm pushing them to the point of fatigue, and the rhythms of my breathing sound like a person stranded in the middle of the ocean without a flotation device. Getting drenched in sweat is awesome, but it means I have to shower another time that day—who has time for that? Going that extra mile feels great in the moment, but it also means I'm limping a little for the remainder of the day from the muscle fatigue. While working out at the gym has its perks, isn't lounging on the couch and watching a movie so much better?

But these days, my love for the gym far outweighs any feelings of slothfulness partly because it is a place where I *feel* so intently. Every time I step into that space I feel the anxious butterflies of middle school me. A few years ago, one of my fitness coaches decided it would be fun to make us pair up with a partner in one of my favorite group fitness classes. I still remember that moment, and I'm not sure I'd been so clammy in all of my adult life. Burpees? Fine. Lunges? Cool. *Finding a partner who wants to be paired with me during a workout?* I'd rather swap out my protein shake with mud. I instantly remembered all those times where I was the last girl picked—for dodgeball, tag, and any other schoolyard activities. I eventually turned into the girl who also felt like the last one picked in love and in life. Our fundamental insecurities have deep roots. For me, as much as the gym is a space of victory, if I'm not careful, it can also turn into a museum of past traumas.

ONE STEP AT A TIME

I distinctly remember one day when I showed up for my group fitness class as I normally did on Friday mornings at 10:15. It was my lucky day because as I was waiting for class to start, a new gym member stood right next to me. Since I'm ever the person who thinks she needs to befriend anyone who so much as breathes the same air as me, I introduced myself. I gave her a few ideas of what to expect during class and assured her that she should relax, have fun, and not worry about doing all the moves perfectly.

As soon as the music started to play, I was in my element. All it takes is the first ten seconds of that loud, semi-chaotic music, and I am filled with adrenaline and ready to leave everything I have on the gym floor. I quickly lost track of my new friend and focused only on my own workout.

Fifty-five minutes later, class was over and she stopped me before I exited the studio. With face red, eyes bloodshot, sweat pouring, and clothes clinging to her body, she said, "Oh my gosh, that was so hard! You are so fit! How did you get through that whole class like it was a breeze?"

After the shock of hearing her words wore off, I smiled

and assured her that it wasn't that long ago that I was the newbie and I, too, thought I'd never get the hang of things. I still remember challenging myself to pursue that very first intense fitness class without letting the size of my body convince me I couldn't.

Just about every time I exercise, I glance back a little.

I think about last year when I got trained to teach my first fitness class—a major milestone that I took on for the sheer goal of proving to myself that I was capable of doing so. But that experience was especially sweet only because of the milestones that I had reached before:

Walking my first mile. After failing many times.

Jogging my first mile. After failing many times.

Running my first mile. After failing many times.

Running my first race. After failing many times.

Running my first nine-miler. After failing many times.

I think one major mind trap in our health and fitness journeys is our future-oriented stance. The whole "set your goals and crush them" dialogue can be a great initial motivator, and goals are good. But sometimes what we really need to do is *look back* at what we've done and where we've come from. When we do, we can give ourselves grace for our journey. Perhaps your body isn't as limber or as tight in some places as you'd like it to be. But look back at your journey and remember the pain and trauma you've carried, the children you've carried, or even just *the burden of life* you've carried. Your body has gotten you through a lot; don't be so hard on it as you strive for whatever change you're reaching for. I remember a time when my body could only take me to the end of the street and back. I reflect on that body with thanks for carrying me then, and I thank my body now for how it carries me through this part of my journey.

My legs have carried me for so many miles. More than I can count. Some days when I look in the mirror, I see them exactly as someone once told me they were . . . huge. I'm tempted to hate them (and some days I fall into that trap). But how can I hate something that has served me so well over the years? And every time I feel the burn deep in my thighs as I do squats or lunges or a long run, I remember once again all the stones I've stepped on to get to where I am today, and I'm filled with gratitude.

Moving your body is an expression of gratitude for how it has been created. Lysa TerKeurst reminds us in her life-changing book that we were *made to crave*.[1] I think we were also *made to move*. But we can walk in true freedom and take another step toward becoming our healthiest selves when we commit to moving our bodies without any fear of judgment (including from ourselves) on their limits. We can easily convince ourselves not to exercise by focusing on the magnitude of what we don't feel capable of doing. What if I had skipped that first walk because I knew I wasn't capable of walking very far? What if I had clung to the thought that the little bit I *could* do wouldn't make a difference? In reality, it was that little bit that made all the difference in my entire journey. It's what got me started, and sometimes that's the hardest part of all.

Exercise is, without a doubt, one of the most vulnerable things we participate in. Nothing about it is comfortable. Sweat in all the places? Had it. So out of breath that I dare not try to speak a word because there's no way someone could understand it? That was me. The *girls* bouncing up and down in chaotic discord because I happened to grab the wrong sports bra? Been there. I've been down the halls of humility and back in my years of exercising, and I will be the first to admit—it isn't easy.

But there's also something about the vulnerability of moving our bodies that, despite it all, is the reason it is so very good for us, in so many ways.

The local YMCA where my family works out has wall-to-wall mirrors in all the fitness rooms. I often get lost in those mirrors. When your identity is so heavily defined by the "before" and "after," it's hard to be fully present in the moment. Being in the space of exercise and fitness forces me to do that. It's the one domain where I can't see myself solely in terms of the past (my failure) or the future (my potential). I have to recognize where I am, here and now—my immediate. Of course, my immediate is defined significantly by who I was and who I want to be. Both are featured prominently in my journey. But in this space, I can't escape into the retreat of "why" (my past) or "when" (my future); I am forced to remain focused on the here and now, which is the "how." Exercise is how I bridge the gap between my past and future.

So much of this book is my attempt to pour something into you, to show you that you are worthy of love, worthy to live life on your own terms, and worthy to care about fitness and health in a way that is meaningful to you and you alone. I invite you to love yourself enough to move, to be vulnerable and open. Look at your past and tip your hat to it. Gaze into the potential of *future* you; she is more powerful and fierce than ever. Give her a good wink to let her know you're on your way. But step back and take a second to appreciate *who you are* in this specific moment in time. See your power and see your potential.

Where you are currently is *enough*. You need to know that. As women, we're constantly in pursuit of *better*. As such, we run on a treadmill of consumerism, always chasing the potential of what could be. This mentality seeps into our exercise journey. We step onto that treadmill, Stairmaster, or rowing machine because we want better abs, arms, and thighs. We buy a dress a size smaller to hang in our closet as a reminder of what we could be. If we're honest with ourselves, most of us are doing work for *future* us.

But what if we change our thinking? What if we shift our focus to care not only for *future us* but also for *present us*—where we are right now? If you get just one thing from this book, I hope it's that. My main goal isn't to get you to change your eating, your fitness routine, or your clothes. I just want you to shift your thinking a bit. What if you could view exercise as something you do not out of obligation but out of love for yourself?

> What if you could view exercise as something you do not out of obligation but out of love for yourself?

I don't need to tell you that exercise is good for you. That is a total duh. You were made to move! It is imperative to your surviving and thriving. It increases physical health as well as emotional health. It reduces the risk of diseases, increases cognitive and emotional capacities, and helps decrease depression and anxiety. Exercise is the closest thing we have to an elixir of youth. It is the catalyst for both *surviving* and *thriving*.

And it has incredible benefits where our emotions and mental health are concerned. When COVID-19 hit and we couldn't go anywhere, I returned to my very first love: walking. We lived in sun-soaked Florida for the first five months of the pandemic, in a neighborhood with miles and miles of sidewalks. Every morning the kids and I would head out for a walk. Then after lunch we found ourselves bored, so out we went again. In the evening, we still had extra time on our hands, so we'd go for yet *another* walk. We did this for days that turned into weeks—then months. It became a part of our everyday life and carried us through many more months of the pandemic, even amid a move north where the sunshine was replaced with snow. We all just felt so much better when we moved our bodies. Our walks became a space to not only get in exercise but to pause, take in nature, talk with each other, hope, dream, and imagine.

It is so easy to neglect the opportunities we have to move our bodies. For so long we've seen exercise as some excruciating hardship we must endure to make our bodies smaller. In that case, it's no wonder we hate it! But there's a better approach.

Just as much as it is our responsibility to love ourselves enough to move our bodies, we also have to recognize that there are legitimate roadblocks. Now's a good opportunity to get vulnerable with yourself and ask, *What are the specific hindrances holding me back from embracing body movement as an enjoyable part of my life?*

LET THE CELEBRATION COMMENCE

For much of my life, I have exercised out of compulsion. I assumed I had to work out if I ever wanted to *lose the weight*— and as I reflect, I'm truly saddened at how much of my health journey has actually been a misguided pursuit to seek out skinny. But skinny as a motivator for exercise does more harm than good. It can be really easy to abandon exercise when it doesn't do what it's "supposed to do." Doing it out of compulsion makes it even harder for us to stay consistent.

Over the years I've leaned into exercise differently. First, I've found that no amount of exercise will ever cause my weight to fluctuate if it isn't paired with fueling my body well. But second, I've come to the conclusion that when I flip the script on how I perceive exercise altogether, my approach is completely different.

These days I view exercise as movement.

We overcomplicate fitness by thinking we have to be marathon runners or gym rats. We see how someone else is working out and think that's our answer too. But what if the right thing for you is something completely unconventional and outside the box? What if while Kiara wakes up at 5:30 a.m. sharp every single day of the week to run her five miles, you sleep in and work in some extra movement throughout your day?

These are the questions we need to ask ourselves when we're constantly hit with the roadblock of not wanting to move our bodies.

I'm going to drop this little truth bomb in your lap so you can free yourself from the pressure to do what you weren't necessarily designed to do: *Your form of movement doesn't have to look like anyone else's.* Neither does your body, your household, your mommying, or anything else. The way you move your body should be specific to what's right for *you*.

Instead of dreading the rigidity of workouts you feel you have to do, what matters is that you find ways to move your body in ways you enjoy. If running isn't your thing, don't run! If the gym isn't your place, don't go! If running around the playground with your kids for thirty minutes suits you better, do that. Simply ask yourself how you can move your body today.

Instead of shaming yourself into moving in uncomfortable ways, celebrate what your body is capable of doing. You parked further away at the grocery store so you could get more steps in—way to go! You worked in some playful squats while you were cooking dinner with your husband tonight—get it, girl! Moving our bodies with joy is exactly how we find consistency so that we can become the very healthiest version of ourselves.

ROADBLOCKS ... WE ALL HAVE THEM!

So let's just say you're ready to start moving that good body of yours, but you're stumbling upon some roadblocks. Not to worry, my friend. Let's take a look at some of the obstacles that try to stop you from living your best life. Identifying the road-blocks that hinder you from moving your body will help you settle into consistency and joy in your healthy-living journey.

I'm just not motivated.

Same here. People who know me know that I exercise a lot. I love the gym, and it's become a part of my daily life, mostly because of the sense of community it brings. But in the spirit of transparency, I have to note that most of the time I don't actually feel like taking that initial step of choosing to work out. Gasp! I know. Most days, I feel like I'm on a collision course, caught between my *will to be fit* and my *desire to just sit*. Women juggle a lot, and between our spouses, kids, jobs, housework, playdates, and everything in between, it's easy to lose motivation to move.

People often ask how I stay motivated. My magic secret isn't such a secret, and I've already shared it in a past chapter— I found my *why*, my ultimate motivation to pursue better health. My *why* pushes me off the couch and into action every time. Because as comfortable as it is to stay in my little resting place, my why is so deeply tattooed onto my heart and mind that I simply cannot revert back to an inactive state of being. I think of my mom, whose physical pain in her own body serves as a reminder to me to never stop moving. I think of my daughter, who has the opportunity to observe good habits and write her story of girlhood and womanhood in a way that is different from mine—free from constant body anxiety. I look at the pile of toys that need picking up, but instead of letting them get in my way, I let them push me to the gym—to help relieve the stress of never feeling like I'm fully caught up and to gain strength to push through household tasks more efficiently in the future.

Think of what exercise and movement are doing for you: clearing your brain, opening up your blood vessels, sending endorphins throughout your body. It took time for me to realize it, but eventually it became clear that no matter how much I might not want to get up and move, I will never, *ever* regret it. And I have also had to realize that my motivation is something I must cultivate regularly. I will always want to find a way out; it's natural because exercise involves growth, and where there is growth, there are growing pains. But finding my *why* helps me clarify my motivation. Find that *why*— whether it is to feel better, keep up with your kids, have more energy, or lower your blood pressure—and I promise you'll find your motivation too.

> *Of course, motivation is not permanent. But then, neither is bathing; but it is something you should do on a regular basis.*
>
> ZIG ZIGLAR

I don't have time.

Time is a hot commodity because we only get a certain amount of it. *Everyone* is pressed for time, and I get that this is a legitimate obstacle. Prioritizing those things that are worthy of our attention can be difficult. By the time we're done with everything we feel like we *have* to do, we're completely spent!

I encourage you, though, not to let this roadblock "win" just because it is legitimate. Time management requires strategic decision-making. There are always things that we must attend to, and there will always be things that we simply can't squeeze in. We have to decide to care enough about ourselves to *make time* to move our bodies.

No matter how busy you are, there's a good chance that you have small pockets of time throughout your day that you could use (or at least add together or reallocate) to allow you to move your body. Can't imagine missing TV time? Consider watching on your phone while you're on the treadmill. Don't want to miss out on a girls' spa day? Take one! But see if the girls want to try a fitness class together sometime. What if you did lunges while doing the dishes? Stretched while doing the laundry? Parked further away from the mall entrance? Volunteered on a class field trip so you could get those extra steps in? Rome wasn't built in a day, and your fitness regime doesn't need to be either. These things take time. Allocating just a bit of *your time* will help you set the stage for future success.

> *Do not wait; the time will never be just right. Start where you stand, and work with whatever tools you may have at your command, and better tools will be found as you go along.*
>
> GEORGE HERBERT

My kids won't let me be great.

Ugh, mine either. While I feel so blessed to be a mother to my beautiful babies, some days it is all I can do to hold myself together as a mommy. My kids, your kids, all kids can be selfish meanies who think of no one but themselves. If you have children, they're the *loves of your life*, but they do take time, energy, and effort. They add so much value, but they also demand a lot.

Many parents let their kids stand in the way of exercise, myself included. I want to always strive for balance. I'd be a liar if I said that there weren't times when my kids won their argument to not go to the gym. Though they love being in the kids' zone with their friends, sometimes they are tired from school and life. I want to model to them that balance is important; rest is just as important as moving; and family is ultimately *more important* than my personal desires. But I also want my kids to know that health takes effort.

I have no easy fix here. (If you've found one, please share it with me.) But one thing our family has done is try to make fitness a core value. Each family member engages in activities that we find fun and meaningful. My husband enjoys intense martial arts–inspired workouts, whereas I like more upbeat, cardio-based fitness classes. My daughter expressed an early interest in running, so we found a local kids' running club to put her in for a mere thirty dollars a year. My son likes jumping from high objects like Superman, so we drape a cape on his shoulders and let him have at it. We solidify *fitness* time and *family* time, all in one. This is one of the reasons we selected our gym—because our kids get to be in the same environment with us, working on their own fitness and personal development while we do the same. We also made sure to select a gym that prioritizes health at every size and not the sort of tight-pants snobbery and he-man groans you might get at other gyms.

If your kids make it hard for you to get regular exercise, try to reimagine how you see family time. It might look different for you than it does for us, but it doesn't need to be elaborate. Never underestimate the value of a simple family walk. Buying family bikes has allowed us to move our bodies together while also teaching our kids valuable lessons about overcoming their fears. My husband and daughter frequently challenge each other to see who can do the most burpees. We've institution-alized fitness into our family dynamic, and it's made us closer.

Our kiddos will likely pose a hindrance to our exercise efforts more times than not, but remember that we're also modeling to them a set of values on health, wellness, and fit-ness. Help shape the next generation in your lineage by incor-porating some of these actions into your core family values. By doing so, you're directly contributing to both the length and quality of your children's lives. Remember, they won't stay little forever. It's okay if your movement looks different in this season of life than it used to or will in the future.

Each day of our lives, we make deposits in
the memory banks of our children.

CHARLES R. SWINDOLL

I feel silly.

Let me tell you one of the best-kept secrets: We all feel silly when we work out. Unless you've been at this for years, it's going to feel vulnerable and awkward. I know what it's like to jiggle when you jump, to have your muffin top spill out over your exercise pants, and to fall completely over when you try to balance. So that you feel better, here's a list of things I have "directly observed" (and never *ever, ever* done myself—this is not about me. Did you get that? It's totally *not* things I've done):

- Slid completely across the gym floor when my sweaty palms slipped while I was doing a "chimp walk." Crashed down in front of others.
- Fell head over heels over the platform in an aerobic step class.
- Toppled down the stairs while trying to run up and down them.
- Dropped a heavy bar in a strength class because I couldn't get it above my head and didn't know what to do.
- Kicked someone (definitely *not* my husband) in a mixed martial arts class.

These are just some of ~~my experiences~~ the experiences I have observed. I could go on and on. I could recount the times that the makeup on my nose completely melted away while the rest of my makeup remained intact, leaving me looking like Rudolph. Or the time I nearly passed out on the treadmill and my husband had to escort me out of the gym before I truly fainted. But there's also the time I literally cried in a workout because I was overcome with appreciation for the fact that my body is capable of doing what I once thought would never be possible.

And so, I persevere. No matter how silly I look, I can't let the opinions of onlookers take up so much space in my decision to do what's best for me.

> *It does not matter how slowly you go so long as you do not stop.*
> CONFUCIUS

I don't have a gym membership.

A gym membership may not be feasible or even desirable for every family. Remember that your fitness is a part of your overall well-being. Breaking the bank and stretching your finances beyond where you're comfortable in order to have a gym membership (which can cost several hundred dollars a month depending on where you live and where you go) does not contribute to that goal. And if you don't live close to a gym, the sheer amount of travel time involved can be a legitimate obstacle.

That said, in our tech-heavy world, a lot is available to you for free. Simply searching YouTube will yield thousands of free workouts you can do at home. Some well-known programs, like Zumba or Les Mills, have primarily paid programming, but even they will have some videos available for free or a reduced price online.

Even if finances aren't a stretch for you, working out at home with free online resources can be a great way to get your feet wet. Imagine wasting hundreds of dollars on a cycle gym membership, only to find that you like hot yoga better. Try your hand at a few things to see what fits you. Search for a jogging group (or start your own), or get together with other women and do some fun movement at the local park. Sign up for a 5K and condition your body to endure it, even if only walking. Go for a family stroll in the evenings. Turn on your favorite music and dance around your house. Whatever works for you.

Once you find what you love, keep pressing forward. Know that many fitness facilities offer reduced memberships to families in need. YMCAs are nationally known for their scholarship programs and (at least in all the Ys I've been a part of) have a policy of never turning any person away due to financial limitations. Exercise is a vulnerable thing, but don't let that vulnerability stop you from moving or from asking for help if you need it. Fitness spaces are community spaces. Find a community that believes in you, and I promise you'll find a community that invests in you.

Obstacles don't have to stop you.
If you run into a wall, don't turn around and give up.
Figure out how to climb it, go through it, or work around it.
MICHAEL JORDAN

I have physical limitations.

While I am an able-bodied person, I am not naive about the fact that so many people carry physical pain or work within the constraints of physical limitations that I do not. This is a legitimate constraint. If you have a physical limitation, step back and evaluate it. In some cases, physical pain is a temporary part of the exercise process. When I began running, my calves would end up super sore the next day . . . but they don't now that my body is conditioned to the form and rhythms of running. When I started lifting, my arms throbbed . . . but they don't now that my muscles have gotten stronger. Exercise can entail some resistance because it's stretching. It's a growing process. And it can be painful at times.

However, if you have physical limitations that are not associated with exercise alone, your best resource is your medical care team. Your health-care providers know your health best and can help you sculpt a meaningful and safe plan of action. Not all exercise is created the same! If high-impact exercise hurts your body, think about swimming. If lifting weights won't work for you, try yoga. There is a litany of options for you out there. And remember, this is your journey. Don't let your inability to do *some of the moves* stop you from participating in the rest. Even in group fitness classes, your instructors and coaches should always be willing to help you make accommodations that fit your own physical needs.

Exercise should be personal—and it can be unconventional. Find what works best for you.

Ultimately, remember that this is *your* journey. You shouldn't apologize for constructing your fitness in a way that makes sense for who you are, where you've come from, what you've been through, and where you want to go.

Nothing stops the man who desires to achieve.
Every obstacle is simply a course to develop his achievement
muscle. It's a strengthening of his powers of accomplishment.

THOMAS CARLYLE

I am exhausted.

If I understand nothing else about your journey, I understand our shared experience of this fact: We are exhausted. I wanted to end with this because (1) it's the reason for not exercising I hear most often, and (2) no matter who you are, if you're reading this, there's a 99 percent chance this phrase applies to you. We run at breakneck speed and juggle a million things. We're tired, overwhelmed, and don't always have the physical or mental energy to do one more thing. And this is where it's important to echo the guiding principle that I hope really defines this whole book: balance.

I want to be clear: It is totally okay to rest. As much as this chapter is about moving your body, it is important to note that your movement will be so much better, faster, stronger, more efficient, and safer if you take time to rest. Life is busy; as much as I truly believe that fitness can be a great outlet to work away the stresses of the world, I also know that being too rigid about our exercise routines will cause us to lose interest and take our focus away from what truly matters. Remember, we aren't doing this to look better; we're doing this to *feel* better. If it feels better to lie on the couch today, take it in stride. We can't lie on the couch all day every day, but if today just isn't your day, try again tomorrow. Pause and ask yourself what your body is telling you it needs, and trust your intuition.

Ultimately, this is about changing our thinking and creating habits that are healthy—and good, healthy habits require balance and honesty.

Whatever you do, keep on moving forward. Put one foot in front of the other. Exercise isn't a "thing" to be achieved; it's not something to be crossed off your to-do list. It isn't something you should put off until later when you actually lose five pounds or when you think you'll be able to succeed. Exercise isn't about succeeding; it's simply about moving. That flies in the face of what we've been conditioned to believe, but you can liberate your mind—and your body—when you see exercise as nothing more than moving wherever you are. Find a way to move your body that is safe, fun, and pushes you forward in life. It's as simple as that.

A man grows most tired when standing still.

CHINESE PROVERB

FINDING A WAY TO MOVE

If you're struggling to find ways to move more, here are some that have worked for me:

- My personal favorite: Try a group fitness class at the gym like BodyPump or a dance class. If this is too intense, try something with less impact, such as a Silver Chair, yoga, or water aerobics class.
- Go for a walk. Just put on some sneakers and get out the door.
- Grab a basketball, soccer ball, or tennis ball and get to a court or field where you can play around for a while.
- Take your kids to the park and chase them around the playground at least half of the time you're there. Remember that you're filling their memory tanks and promoting the value of physical fitness.
- Search for "workouts to do at home" on YouTube or Pinterest. RevWell TV and Fitness Blender are also great resources and have hundreds of videos that stream for free.
- Call a local gym near you and see if they offer a free trial or a visitor's choice. Show up and try it! You might love it.
- Go for a run or jog. Feel the wind on your face and pace yourself so you don't overdo it. If it gets to be too much, take it down to a walk. Soak up nature!

- Find a set of stairs in your community or somewhere in your town. Run or walk up and down them as many times as you can.
- Sit on the floor and stretch your body.
- Do the basics. Set a timer for twenty minutes and do some standard exercises like jumping jacks, push-ups (knees or toes!), crunches, burpees, squats, lunges, or high-knee running in place.
- Turn on some fun music and dance as vigorously as you can while you clean your house.
- Park in the farthest parking space whenever you go somewhere this week.
- Try a boxing class or some other program you've always wanted to try.
- Pull out your bike (or rent a bike if you don't have one) and go for a long ride.
- Head to a community pool, the pool at your gym, or the pool in your backyard. Try doing something you don't normally do, like swimming underwater or swimming laps. And remember, no one cares how you look in a swimsuit. It's in your head. Jump in that water, girl. Cannonball if you'd like!
- Go shopping. This keeps you on your feet, and if you go all day, you'll get a lot of steps in without even thinking about it. (Please note, my husband does not endorse this option.)
- Mow the lawn or do yard work.
- Do squats while folding the laundry.

- Get up and move while you're watching TV.
- In the kitchen, move your arms in different ways while waiting for food to cook.

MORE THAN YOU THINK YOU CAN

We're all guilty of placing limits on ourselves. The biggest obstacles we face are ideas: ideas about our self-worth, our determination, and our abilities. When I first started moving my body, I constantly thought about how it was nearly impossible for me. It hurt and it wasn't fun. I didn't think I'd ever be able to do anything athletic, I didn't think I could stick with exercise, and I wasn't sure it was worth it.

But now it feels good. And it often lifts my spirits like nothing else can.

I can tell you *exactly* how I bridged that gap—by putting one foot in front of the other, each time just one step further. Fatigue set in every time, as it will. And each time I quietly whispered to my fatigue that I wasn't giving up. I pushed past the urge to quit and got a little stronger. Suddenly that quarter-of-a-mile walk down the road turned into a mile, then two, then a 5K. I kept going and going, but none of it happened overnight. And it didn't start with a run or even a light jog; it started with a mindset.

While running isn't my all-time favorite exercise, I do enjoy it occasionally. When my shoes find that steady rhythm and the air fills my lungs and wind makes the trees dance as if they're cheering me on, I feel empowered with every stride, no matter the distance I go that day. I head out the door with no expectations of mileage or speed, and I just lean into the moment as my strong legs carry me farther and farther.

A few months ago I headed out the door, announcing to Phil that I was going to run a couple of miles. A while later I sent him a text that said, "Four miles in, just a couple more and I'll be home shortly!" When I finally walked through the front door with tears in my eyes, I held up nine fingers. I had slowly and steadily put one foot in front of the other and run the farthest I'd ever run. I wasn't motivated by the number, or the hope that I'd weigh less the next morning, or the fact that I torturously pushed through some workout I hated. It was my frame of mind that carried me through every one of those nine miles.

It was a hundred times of saying in my heart, in my head, and even out loud, "Yes, you can, Jennifer." It was the flashbacks to 336-pound me that would have given anything for the physical capability to run like that. It was the fact that stopping would have been fine at any moment and that I actually enjoyed challenging myself to give my best. Whatever my best was that day.

We're often told that "if we can think it, we can do it." That sounds good, but it can be limiting. We can actually do a lot *more* than we think we can—we just have to start seeing ourselves as capable. We often reduce our abilities based on low self-esteem, self-doubt, or bad past experiences. While our bodies have limits and we need to respect our

> We can actually do a lot *more* than we think we can—we just have to start seeing ourselves as capable.

health, life is about growth. Pushing past your comfort zone is empowering and changes the dynamics of fitness. Instead of you against the world (falling prey to the comparison trap we've talked about), it's now you versus you. This is a way to take charge and take control of your health journey. You call the shots, you make the rules, and you set the goal.

Regular movement is a fundamental step in your health journey and a way to celebrate that your body is good. Remember, no matter what kind of movement you pursue—whether it's a stroll down the street or a triathlon, *you can do it.* Now the question is, *how will you move your body today?*

Flip the Script

Instead of telling yourself, "I'm too big to move like that," say this instead: **"Exercise is a celebration of what my body is capable of, and I can move in ways I enjoy."**

Reflect

What past experiences have affected your view of exercise? How could thinking about movement rather than exercise change your perspective?

Action Step

Pause, stand up, ask Alexa to play a song you can dance to, and dance around the room. Take notice of how good it feels to get your blood flowing, your lungs taking full breaths, and your body moving.

Chapter 8

YOU DESERVE TO EAT

Pizza, Ben and Jerry, and I had one *last* meeting before we were (actually . . . really . . . honestly this time) breaking it off for good. We were cuddled up on the couch like high school sweethearts waiting for our parents to come home—knowing we shouldn't be so close but also fully aware that we were far more attached than met the eye.

If someone was writing my life story, that's how it might begin. I love food. I write about it, talk about it, think about it, experiment with it—endlessly. I've come to realize that food plays an important role in our journeys. And truthfully, its role for many can be just as much emotional as it is physical.

Pizza is a comfort food for me. It goes back to my teen-age years. We were poor—like *poor* poor—and could rarely afford to eat out. The food stamps we got only covered so much, and within a house where my mom struggled to get by, the food we ate regularly was not exactly Gordon Ramsey–approved.

Food is communal. Emotional. *Powerful.*

But once in a while, the heavens would open up and my mom would go out and buy pizza from Domino's or Papa John's. Though my palate has now elevated to a strict New York-style pizza only, *thankyouverymuch,* back then that pizza brought a comfort that was often lacking in our house. It might seem ridiculous to you as you read this, but pizza was the only hope we had. We yearned for it because it meant that we weren't "struggling" in that moment. And when we got it, I felt like the little orphan Annie who had just struck it big with Daddy Warbucks.

Before you roll your eyes at my melodrama, I want to challenge you to step back and think about a food from your childhood that makes you feel happy or cared for. It was probably a family staple, and I'm guessing it wasn't celery and hummus.

Food is communal. Emotional. *Powerful.*

But food also has an enemy—a four-letter word that stands ready to police it, keeping it from having its way with us with abandon. A mortal enemy so savage that it seeks to steal every ounce of joy that food has by starving it out of existence.

I'm talking, of course, about our good friend *Mr. Diet.* He isn't any normal mister, either. He's a CEO of a multibillion-dollar company. Though it's hard to wrap our heads around the number, estimates point to the weight-loss and diet market in the United States as a more than $72 billion-dollar industry.[1] That diet mindset that we think about constantly, the one we'll try on for size again after the holidays or as we gear up for swimsuit season? It's no harmless thought network; it's a robust, financially staggering industry that seeks to devour us in a sea of promised results, magic pills, and newly discovered formulas.

Now let me be clear, adopting a new approach to eating that includes trusting your intuition and incorporating a variety of foods and nutritional sources is good for you. But being *on a diet?* Not so much. In our Western society, we quickly associate "diet" with a set of restrictions on our food intake that are unachievable at best, dangerous at worst. Sure, there is scientific data to back up why we should monitor what goes in our mouths; we want to avoid negative substances such as excess sodium, processed fats, and chemicals. These are legitimate concerns. After all, your body is a temple—you probably shouldn't wash its stained-glass windows with turpentine.

But when it comes to diets, let's be serious—many of us (particularly women) don't "watch what we eat" for fear of ingesting carcinogens or raising our cholesterol. We do so out of fear of what the scale tells us. We'll survive for a few weeks (or days) on chickpeas and cucumbers. But eventually, when our body rightfully tells us that we're being crazy, we don't know how to regulate so we're right back to where we started with Ben, Jerry, and Colonel Sanders (don't judge me—we all have our issues).

Changing the way we eat is no easy task because we've been eating the way we've been eating for a really long time. Throughout our lifespans we've been developing what are now our daily habits and mindsets about food. My husband grew up in the mountains of Pennsylvania in a tiny Dutch-German-Amish community. When I met the guy, he'd literally never heard of asparagus. And broccoli was what you put in a casserole smothered in cheese. Food is such a part of our family narratives and communal lives. As our palates evolve, food becomes part of our overall identity. Food isn't just food—it's a part of who we are and how we understand the world.

When my grandmother discovered that cancer had consumed nearly her entire body, friends and family urged her to switch to a completely plant-based lifestyle. She wasn't necessarily *opposed* to doing that, but she had been eating a certain way for seventy years. Those foods contained the comfort of childhood familiarity. She *wanted* to be healthy. She didn't *want* to have cancer. She *believed* that eating a plant-based diet (or at least one free of known cancer aggravators) could possibly help her condition. But her Southern Ozark cooking was, in many ways, the only comfort, familiarity, and stability she had as the rest of her life, health, wellness, and mortality all seemed to be called into question.

This is one major reason dieting is not a great method for journeying toward our healthiest selves. Because in its simplest form, a diet is basically pressure to completely change your way of eating. But the idea of undergoing an overhaul in our eating habits is overwhelming. We don't want to give up the foods we love; even *if* and *when* we're willing to, it's often after an emotional breakdown, and we doubt our ability to stick to our new eating plan. We hold tight to the doctrine of "all or nothing." Though we know it's complete bunk, we subscribe to a philosophy that is crippling to our lives and our health: that we must either (1) dive into a strict, restrictive diet program devoid of all food that tastes good and gives us joy or (2) keep eating the way we're eating and hope that one day we'll have what it takes to make "the change."

But this "change" is not permanent. There's *nothing* permanent about our health and wellness journeys. As we'll talk about later in chapter 9, we're virtually always in process, somewhere in the middle of our journeys. We forget this when we fall prey to the idea that one "mistake" is an indictment of our ability. So in our feelings of incapability we shove two handfuls of M&M's into our mouths to ease the sting. And instead of enjoying those sweet little beauties as the amazingness they are, we internally scorn ourselves for what we perceive as a failure. I mean, how often have you heard (or said) phrases like:

I've got to get back on the bandwagon.
I cheated a bit today.
I messed up. I'll start again Monday.

Sound familiar? Oh, yes. For me too. Been there, done that, got the stretch marks to prove it.

MY MOST EXTREME DIETING EXCURSION

Throughout my crazy, roller-coaster journey of weight loss, I have tried nearly every diet you can imagine. My life has been all but cosponsored by the diet industry. Weight Watchers, keto, veganism, vegetarianism, Adkins, Paleo, Trim Healthy Mama, ten-day smoothie cleanses, don't eat after 4 p.m. but do the hokey-pokey at 6 p.m. sharp . . .

When I tell you I've done it all, I've done it all.

But none of these diets "work." Why? Because all of them work. Temporarily. That's their design. Like a relationship with a high school sweetheart, the relationship you have with these diets was never meant to last forever. While a small handful of programs out there center on weight loss *without* dieting (good news, that's a thing!), most are a straight shot to the downward spiral of failure we all dread.

Perhaps the craziest of all the crazy diets I've tried involved taking a hormone typically associated with pregnancy: HCG. I quiver as I type those three letters. I had seen a well-known influencer boasting on social media about her super-fast weight-loss experience, and in my post-baby desperation after my daughter was born, I was intrigued. Her results seemed undeniable. Day after day, I saw her before-and-after snapshots flash across my newsfeed, and finally, in a moment of despair, I decided to give her method a try. By that point, I had failed so many times that I was actively considering bariatric surgery to help me. (Side note: I do not mean to belittle bariatric surgery. People choose this route for a variety of reasons.) That first 100 pounds I'd lost years before in my initial push had seemed to glide off my body, but since then it felt like nothing was getting me closer to the weight-loss goals I had my sights set on. Every time I tried to jump back on the bandwagon something threw me off again. I decided that HCG would be my final attempt before I went the surgery route.

The HCG diet was "simple," the doctor who prescribed it assured me. I'd simply come to visit the physician every week for a B-12 shot. That's because my immune system would be suppressed due to a lack of nutrition that I'd normally acquire through food. Between those weekly doctor visits, I'd be injecting a synthetic version of the human growth hormone into myself every single day, twice a day, for six weeks. With a needle. Oh, and I forgot to mention, I could only eat 500 calories a day maximum, with very strict restrictions on how those calories could be consumed. "No cheating allowed," I was warned. Even one cheat or extra indulgence and the HCG could actually work *the opposite way*, making me gain weight. Oh, and it was expensive.

Simple, right? It wasn't. Those six weeks were utter agony. You don't realize the role food plays until it's absent from your life. I'm not only talking about an unhealthy attachment to food here; I'm talking about sustenance, feeling "full" or satisfied, and simply feeling like you have the fuel to get through life. Sure, I lost weight—how could I not? But much of it crept back on after the six weeks were done, and the diet had a long-term negative effect on my metabolism, one that has taken years to overwrite. In fact, the doctor who prescribed HCG to me swore off the method shortly afterward because she observed the profound long-term effects were far worse on the human body than a couple of extra pounds.

Don't do this. I beg you. I understand the weight struggle. But as pressing as it may seem to drop pounds, it's harder to drop them through extreme and unhealthy changes, only to gain them back. Sure, you'll lose weight, but the toll these quick-fix diets take on your body will leave you in a worse condition than when you started. The number on the scale went down thanks to the HCG diet, but so did my muscle mass, my mood, my metabolism, my sex drive, and my joy for life. Did I shed a few pounds? Yes. Did I develop a healthy perspective about eating? No. Did I find balance? No. Did I feel the freedom to enjoy food and eating? No.

In fact, I never realized that last feeling was possible. By this point in my life, I had become a platinum member of the lifetime Yo-Yo Dieting Club. I only knew the polar extremes of excess—excess eating and food consumption or excess dieting and restriction. Neither end of this spectrum held joy. It wasn't joyful to restrict my eating, and honestly, it wasn't joyful to gorge on cake. Both were just part of the rhythm that I had accepted as normal.

That cadence is not sustainable because it doesn't

produce balance. And if you are not embracing your health journey as one of balance and consistency, you are setting yourself up to fail. Any positive results you experience will only be short-term.

WHO WEARS THE PANTS?

Ultimately, our success in life comes down to our relationships. It's hard to have a successful marriage without a good relationship with your partner. It's hard to succeed in the world of work if you don't have a good relationship with your boss. So ask yourself what magical powers you think you have that will cause you to be healthy and well if you don't have the right relationship with food.

Think of food as a person. You interact with it every single day—in fact, you have a physiological date with it every few hours. You need it. You crave it, almost like you crave time with your significant other. This is normal.

But normal can quickly become perverse if it's not held to a standard of accountability. When we depend on something, it has the power to keep us in bondage. In romantic relationships, this is less of an issue since we expect our significant other to have our best interests in mind. Not true of food. We're in a relationship with it, but it doesn't care about us. If we're not careful, food can trick us into thinking we have no control. It features so prominently in our day-to-day lives that our relationship with it becomes mindless and unregulated. But like all other relationships, if no one is putting forth the effort to see that relationship blossom in a healthy way, it will fail.

And unlike that guy you dated for 4.25 seconds in college, food doesn't just disappear from your life. Even if you try to break up, you have to keep interacting with it no matter what.

I want you to understand that *the way you see food* is more important than the details of every bite that enters your mouth. That's what will cause you to succeed in this area of your life. And here's the thing: The quality of the relationship we have with food is solely and completely up to us. Do we have control over it, or does it have control over us? When we can negotiate the power in this relationship, we can start to pursue healthy eating in a way that is empowering and *healthy.*

I refuse to live in bondage to food. I refuse to let food (or the pressure to be on a diet) have power over me. I'm calling the shots here. I wear the pants in this relationship and yes, on some days they might be my *stretchy* pants, but I'm still the one in charge.

FINDING FOOD FREEDOM

In dieting, as in many aspects of life and culture, there's a pendulum that swings left and right, driving the rhythm, including our mindset about food. When the pendulum swings too far, we often rely on extreme means to overcorrect. Too far toward *restriction* and we're miserable, so we swing the other way toward *excess.* Too far toward *excess* and we're miserable again. This is the drastic pattern that I found myself in for most of my life. As I've worked on my relationship with food, I've found a reduced range of motion on the pendulum, and that has allowed me to walk toward food freedom.

My goal here is not to give you detailed guidance on nutrition or how to eat to lose weight. While I've spent some time in the past trying to help women approach weight loss in a healthy way, I now prefer to educate people on finding freedom in their health journey. I look back at some of my former blog entries that focus on weight loss as a primary goal and see how much farther I've come in my own journey to freedom. I spent so many years trying to nail down to a science every single bite of food I put into my mouth. To this day my stomach turns when someone says the words "steamed broccoli" because I ate it hundreds of times, day after day, week after week, year after year, trying to lose weight. Bleh.

Nowadays I'm working really hard to learn how to eat intuitively. Sometimes I close my eyes, take a breath, and take a second to think, *What am I actually hungry for right now?* I'm learning to trust my intuition and the fact that my body will give me clues as to what it needs. This process has been incredibly freeing, but it didn't happen overnight. Learning to eat intuitively takes practice, trial and error, and that lovely thing we all love to hate: T.I.M.E. But I can assure you that it is worth it.

Intuitive eating starts with the realization that you

> Your food choices are not attached to your personal character, so there is no need to agonize over whether every bite of food is "right."

deserve to eat without guilt and shame. Your food choices are not attached to your personal character, so there is no need to agonize over whether every bite of food is "right." From there, give yourself permission to explore a reality in which you trust your gut when it comes to eating. This doesn't mean you'll magically begin to nourish your body with ease, but it does mean that you can ask yourself questions about what your body needs in any given moment. This will help you honor your hunger and the cues your body gives you when it needs something. It will also allow you to truly enjoy that delicious something you used to think of as a "cheat" and will eventually bring new waves of self-confidence and freedom in your eating habits. Remember, the goal isn't to ease our way right back to diet culture, where we're only eating carrot sticks and grilled chicken. The goal is to embrace and enjoy a wide variety of foods and learn how to fuel our bodies so we can feel our absolute best.

It's amazing when an apple is just an apple. A scoop of ice cream is just a scoop of ice cream. A few bites of Moses' mac and cheese is . . . you get the drift. A cookie is not a cheat, an act of greed or gluttony, a slip-up, or a bad choice. It's just a cookie. As I practice this more and more, I find that beautiful balance in which the pendulum is not thrusting me toward misery. That, my friend, is freedom.

If this isn't a nutrition chapter, what is it? I'd argue that it's a *freedom* chapter. Freedom is where stability, normalcy, consistency, and peace lie, and it's what most of us are searching for. When it comes to food, what if instead of feeling bewildered as the pendulum swings from side to side, we take things one decision at a time? What if instead of seeing bread as a failure and hummus as a success, we learn that the most accurate and healthy picture of wellness will most likely include *both of those*?

Contrary to popular belief, your kryptonite isn't carbs—it's self-doubt and guilt. When we swing between restriction and excess, those extremes become our normal. My "normal" has been me being down on myself, doubting my ability to make healthy choices, and then feeling guilty for making an "eating error." I now realize that's because I have strived for perfection, which in reality is unattainable. I have failed in this journey because I wanted an outcome that isn't even possible. There isn't a simple, static outcome at the end of my journey because my journey doesn't end—it simply continues on. It's a process.

My kids love to play *Mario Kart* on their gaming devices. They are both terrible at it (don't tell them I said that), and I know that because they are constantly driving off the side of the road, effectively ending their rounds. What happens? The game shuts down, they "lose a life," and the round starts over. That's how we've approached the health journey. We get "off course" and boom—we lose a life (or at least our minds) and then we think we have to start all over. But if we stopped seeing our food choices as a test of whether we're strong enough to make the "right" decision, we'll see that life and health and wellness might include everything from cauliflower to cake pops.

This trips up a lot of people. They want a "quick fix," which means they want a list of foods to eat and foods to avoid, plus a designated point where they should stop and start. Now don't hate me when I bring the bad news, but this wellness journey has no stopping point. On the one hand, I understand how that can be discouraging, particularly because we are such goal- and destination-oriented people. But on the other hand, for those of us who really, *really* want to finally be comfortable living an ongoing healthy life, this can actually be encouraging. It means that nothing—no food choice, no eating plan, no weight gain or loss—is the be-all and end-all! Seeing our health journey as an ongoing process eliminates guilt. We don't have to or even get to "start over" after a food indulgence; we just take it for what it is—one choice in a lifetime of an infinite number of choices—and keep moving forward.

WORK IT, GIRL (YOUR WILLPOWER, THAT IS . . .)

Start. Fail. Repeat.

This is the bread and butter of the diet industry. Marketers bank on our failures and know the emotional toll that comes along with them. They bank on our limited storehouse of willpower as we gear up for a diet, knowing good and well it will eventually run out. They know that after we get desperate enough again (and we will), we'll come crawling back, probably spending more money, trying even harder to succeed.

Take that bread and butter back from the diet industry, put it in the toaster, and have it for breakfast instead. Instead of putting your willpower and trust behind some diet, put that willpower and trust in your own abilities to make the choices that will further your overall wellness. Instead of leaning on willpower to carry you toward food freedom, try taking things one decision at a time.

Every single time you choose what is right for you in that moment, you prove to yourself once again that you can trust your intuition for what your body needs. Over time, making those right choices becomes easier. If you're one of the millions of us who struggle to nourish our bodies in a way that is free from diet culture, let me give you a few little pointers that I use sometimes.

Rome wasn't built in a day. Start small.

I have to repeatedly remind myself that I didn't get to my breaking point overnight. My rock-bottom moment happened after years of trauma, disordered eating, and turning to food for comfort in an uncomfortable life. Those experiences etched themselves deeply onto my body, and ridding myself of them won't happen immediately.

But frankly, I don't even want to rid myself completely of those experiences. They were hard, but they shaped me. I've learned in my long, slow journey of health and fitness that even bad past experiences can continue to teach me about myself.

By going slow, I allow myself to sit with discomfort. Each day when I look in the mirror, I don't see the butterfly; I see the caterpillar she once was. But I don't see only the trauma and hurt either; I see a resilient woman who has overcome on her own terms and in her own way, one small change at a time. Starting small is a critical component of success in all of the areas we've discussed in this book—how we view our bodies and deal with the pressure to be perfect, how we develop the right motivation, and how we approach movement and think about food.

Small progress is still *progress*. If you take the time to process one small decision, following through can build your confidence quickly. In the context of fueling our bodies, small progress might mean eating an extra bite or two of fresh produce today. Small but significant!

I'm not a certified nutritionist, so please be sure that *your* small changes fit with your larger goals and health plan. Someone who is trying to lower blood pressure to increase energy may need to make different choices than someone who is trying to avoid spikes and dips in blood sugar every day. But no matter the goal, start small and acknowledge the progress you've made. Instead of trying to shed the pounds or shed the past, shed the idea that your identity is wrapped up in a "before and after" and then journey toward the healthiest you.

Put off for tomorrow what will make you stronger today

Some of us, instead of completely depriving ourselves, need to give ourselves space to practice patience. Learning to hold off for a little while can be helpful as long as it doesn't send us into a deprivation deep dive. We've been told that we have to learn to say no, but what if that was a lie? What if sometimes instead of no, the better answer is, "Maybe later, but not right now"?

As you know by now, I've got an incessant sweet tooth and my blood type is Pepperoni+. While I'd love to have pizza and ice cream every single night, that would probably not lead to me feeling nourished and free. So instead of telling myself no for as many days in a row as I possibly can, I simply work these foods into our regular eating habits. I've found that this allows me to trust my decision on when to order pizza for dinner or take the kids out for ice cream. I don't feel like I'm constantly avoiding these foods, or that I have to muster up the world's strongest willpower muscle to say no yet *again*.

It's okay to order a pizza. It's okay to hold off until tomorrow. It's also okay to trust your decision.

Be mindful in the moment

Our minds are so easily distracted. It takes little to nothing for me to find myself scrolling my phone mindlessly for hours on end. My kids can be screaming in the next room, but with the entire digital world at my fingertips, I might as well be in Bora Bora.

Food often plays a part in our daily mindlessness. We slip our hands into a bag of chips or find a spoonful of ice cream in our mouths as we reflect on the troubles of the day. But what happens when we turn our mindlessness into mindfulness?

Mindful eating happens when we give our attention to what we're eating while we're eating it. We're not thinking of what's to come or what was but rather what's happening in this very moment. This can help us inch our way toward food freedom, as it allows us to fully enjoy what we're consuming.

I've started asking myself questions like:

- What sounds yummy to you?
- Are you enjoying that plate of food?
- Do you wish you were eating something else?
- How does it taste or smell?
- How does it leave you feeling after you're finished eating it? Full? Satisfied? Energized?

By doing this, I've been more capable of listening to my body's hunger cues, needs, and yes, even determining what my body *wants!*

Stress less to avoid the mess

I'm a mom of two, and I get stressed a lot. My sister is a mom of eleven and gets stressed a lot. Some of my friends have no kids, and guess what? They're stressed too! The world we live in is complex, dynamic, ever-expanding, and changing, and it can be exhausting to keep up with. Stress is a part of all our lives, and when we're stressed, it's tough to make mindful food choices. We just don't have the energy, so we get lost in whatever falls into place.

When we're stressed, our cortisol levels increase, which leads to increased cravings (often for high-carb foods, as carbs help to decrease cortisol levels). But if we train our bodies to use food as our only go-to stress release, then we're pushing ourselves into a cycle of defeat that can lead to feeling out of control. Yes, you totally could indulge in a candy bar from the work vending machine on those days when your boss gets a little crabby. I vote yes. Do that sometimes. But you may also find that a better way to deal with the stress is to give yourself a chance to breathe, talk, cry, or some other thing that will not cause a sugar crash in a couple of hours.

No matter how you deal with stress, be present in the moment, paying attention to what is happening right now. Emotions are sometimes attached to the food choices we make, and that's not always the worst thing in the world. Sometimes you just need to throw your home-cooked dinner plans out the window and go eat at your favorite restaurant. It is what it is. But no matter what you do, being attentive to your emotions will help you deal with stress the way that's right for you.

Make a plan, Stan

In the season of life I find myself in, social gatherings reinforce my love of community and connectedness. But those gatherings often involve foods and beverages that for many years had a stronghold in my life. It is tough to be in a situation where we feel like we have to choose a healthy alternative over a yummy or fun one. Not to mention feeling pressure to eat (or not eat) certain things. In a space where we should be having fun and letting loose, we're consumed with a thousand different thoughts about what everyone else wants us to do. This is where taking a moment to plan our approach might help.

Remember, you don't *have to* eat the salad and you don't *have to* forgo the chocolate cake. You can choose. No, really— *you get to choose*. Remove yourself for a moment from every opinion and every *should* and do what works best for you.

Are you headed to a family function where people will make comments about your food choices? Are you feeling pressure to eat or avoid certain foods simply to appease other people (or even *yourself*)? The choices you make should lie in your own hands because you are capable of making your own decisions on what you eat.

Make a plan for how you'll handle these things in a way that keeps you true to you. This way you're not derailed in the moment.

FOOD IS A GOOD THING

Growing up, and into my early adult years, my food habits were . . . how should I put this . . . complete and utter garbage. Part of this goes back to my roots. In my family, you were either on a diet of vegetable soup and green apples or you were gorging like your life depended on it. It's important for me to be able to admit that I was out of control—that recognition helps drive me toward balance today. I'm talking upsized everything, candy before/during/after every meal. If the thought of a snack popped into my head, I got it and ate it. Food was a coping mechanism for the ongoing trauma I was experiencing over the course of my entire childhood and teenage years.

Food has always been my escape. It's that way sometimes, isn't it? Life becomes a whirlwind, our heads are spinning, and we don't know backward from forward. Things get fuzzy and out of focus. Nothing seems concrete. At least that's how I have felt *many* times throughout my life. Especially growing up. I had no control over where I lived, where I went to school, or how I would make friends in a new place, but I *did* have a degree of control over what I ate. Food became my emotion-regulator, my de-stressor, and my comfort. Food was the only security I knew. When you combine that with having divorced parents, moving around all the time, poverty, and generational struggles with health and wellness, it's no wonder I found myself in so much bondage to food.

Food has had power over me for most of my life. And to be extremely honest, in some ways it still does. I write this chapter for me as much as I write it for you. We're learning together. But what changed my relationship with food was changing the way I thought about it.

Instead of seeing food as a means to losing weight, I started to see food as *fuel*. As *nourishment*. As a *good* thing.

The foods we eat (and how *much* we eat of them) dictate how our bodies function. As I paid more attention to the correlation between how I was fueling my body and how my body felt, I began to crave nourishment above eating for reduced pounds on the scale. When I realized that drinking a big glass of water gives me a burst of energy a mere twenty minutes later, hydration became more important to me. When incorporating protein into every meal quieted my hunger pangs, I started building my meals differently. When eating carbs and fats steadied my blood sugar and decreased my headaches, I was more open to learning how to incorporate them into my daily diet. When I finally woke up to the fact that gigantic portions left me feeling physically and emotionally worn down every single time, I stopped pushing past the point of being satisfied when I ate.

Our bodies deserve good fuel because we love them, because food is amazing, and because they do a lot of work carrying us through life every day. When we lean into food as a good thing, we can be less ruled by our emotional waves and more guided by our intuition about what our bodies need in any given moment. This is how we walk toward food *freedom*—no longer bound to food in a way that dictates our choices out of fear.

FOOD FOR THOUGHT

I'm most certainly not a nutritionist, but I like to share these very basic keys that have helped me along this massive journey of mine. Do I have all of this figured out? No way. My journey will always keep evolving, and I will forever continue learning. My simple way of navigating the world of food, diets, and the empty promises that come with them is to uphold three basic standards for my eating.

- **Is it doable?** Can this be done over time, in nearly any space or place? Is it sustainable in the daily ups and downs of life? Does it require effort (okay) but not anguish (not okay)?

- **Is it healthy?** Does it focus not just on how much and what we eat but on our overall relationship with food and moving our bodies? Or does it promise something that seems too good to be true? Because, hon, these diet companies be lyin' to ya.
- **Is it balanced?** Will it allow you to enjoy the foods you love while giving you the freedom to follow your own intuition for what your body needs? Does it incorporate every food group (of course, making adjustments based on your own individual life circumstances) without crossing off things like bread and even sweets?

No diet company will give you that holy trinity of advice because it can't be sold. But if you follow those three principles—ensuring that you're also feeding your *inner being* with the right food and messages—you'll find yourself walking toward freedom in no time.

This entire book is about loving your body and remembering that it is *good*. Learning to love your body doesn't mean throwing *who you are and the things you enjoy* out the window the moment you decide to pursue a healthier life. And it also doesn't mean ditching all your health goals the moment you fail. Loving yourself the way you are means that you value yourself enough—here and now with no strings attached—to be mindful, purposeful, and intentional about your journey. Learning to love your body allows you to break the bondage that diets and food have had over you and instead reclaim your story on your own terms. It means finding as much satisfaction in the baby steps as in the pounds lost and as much satisfaction in the brownie after date night as in the intentional and mindful choice you made by ordering the salad instead of the fries.

Learn that you have what it takes to conquer in this area of your life. Grab on to the food pendulum with both hands to stop it from swinging to the two extremes. Demand that balance and freedom define this journey for you.

Flip the Script

Instead of telling yourself, "I need to go on a diet," say this instead: **"I can remove guilt and embrace mindfulness and freedom in my food choices."**

Reflect

Consider your relationship with food. How did events in your childhood shape some of your thought patterns about food? How could your relationship with food change if you walked toward food freedom and intuitive eating instead of restrictive dieting?

Action Step

Think about a food-related scenario that comes up frequently in your life, like being stressed after a bad work call or coming home famished after a long day. Jot down three ways you can practice food freedom in this moment.

Chapter 9

WELCOMING THE MIDDLE

There's a sort of running joke that I've heard people make when they look at old pictures of themselves: "If I was as skinny now as I was back then when I thought I was fat . . ." I *feel* that joke in my core because it has held true during so many seasons of body change in my life. Much like we've come to expect to see bodies as digitally altered artifacts, so, too, have we come to see bodies in terms of *before* and *after*. But no good story has just a beginning and an end. The real meat and bones is found in the *middle*. That's where the enjoyable part of the journey takes place.

In our body journeys, it is easy to forget that there's a middle. Because we're always pursuing an after, we forget that we're living in the middle, right here and right now.

I can hardly stand to admit this, but I have spent the majority of my life trying to lose weight, constantly striving for yet another after photo, even when I'd already reached a goal. As I've matured and reflected, I've realized that I didn't know what it felt like *not* to be consumed with losing weight because that had been a never-ending journey for me. I always figured that once I hit my goal weight, I could stop the tug-of-war in my brain and finally just go to a restaurant, eat what sounded good, and leave feeling satisfied but not stuffed. But I never reached that point.

For the entire year after that night years ago when I reached my breaking point, weight loss was steady. It was a daily decision to wake up and check off all the weight-loss action items. At the time I hadn't met Phil yet, and I didn't have little ones running around demanding every ounce of my time, energy, and focus. It was just Jennifer focusing on Jennifer. Things were still up and down, but generally headed in the right direction.

After a year (and 100 pounds) down, things went wonky. I stepped into a stressful job, went back to school full-time, and met the love of my life. It was a whirlwind of juggling my big-girl job, studying for exams, and being completely smitten. My decision-maker was fatigued, and it was hard remembering to eat the right things, finding time to exercise, and staying consistent. My habits were much healthier than they'd been earlier in my life, but now that I wasn't hyperfocused on losing weight, the scale didn't budge.

I assumed that things would slow down and I could get

back on track. But . . . nope. Next came marriage and a baby in the baby carriage and a big move halfway across the country (to Kansas, where the only thing to do is watch the corn grow . . . and eat), and an even more stressful job. Before I knew it, a few years had passed and I was still lingering in the 100-pounds-lost club. I actively worked to continue the momentum of weight loss that I'd experienced initially, but nothing seemed to bring the results I wanted.

It took about five years of trying to lose weight but staying stagnant for me to understand that while I was constantly reaching for an end point, I was completely neglecting the joy of being in the middle of the journey.

WHAT IS THE MIDDLE?

Moving around a lot the way I did as a child came with its challenges, but one major advantage is that I've been able to see a lot of the United States and appreciate beauty in a variety of locations. My all-time favorite place, though? Tennessee. I have such nostalgic memories of a treasured family trip we took there when I was a child. We drove through the mountains and past cascading streams and rivers. To me, Tennessee provides serenity and a sense of calm like no other place on earth. It is the one spot I can hear myself think, move, and breathe. It was halfway between our journey from South Florida to Michigan (a trip we made several times in order to visit my dad), and I always looked forward to reaching that midpoint in the journey. In that space and place, I was fully content to be lost in the middle of nowhere.

But I don't want just any old middle of nowhere. My husband grew up in a town almost isolated from all outside human contact, buried between two ridges in Central Pennsylvania. Though I've grown to love our visits there, I didn't always love taking the trek up the mountains to the woods that Phil calls home. Why? Because *that* middle of nowhere is different from the one I'm comfortable with. There are bears (Seriously! My husband has a great tale of almost hitting one with his car as a teenager), coyotes, snakes of all types, porcupines, skunks, and all the other animals that make those sounds you hear in scary movies set deep within the woods. I'm no princess, but I'm also no cave woman.

By its definition, the *middle* is "equally distant from the extremes of our limits."[1] The spaces I mentioned above are intentionally isolated. Their whole identity is staked on being *away*—away from big cities, loud traffic, and human interruption. Whether we see their beauty immediately in the landscape of Tennessee's Smoky Mountains or have to *learn* how to love them, like driving up the huge mountain to Beaver Springs, Pennsylvania, both have the same purpose. And we can shift our thinking and find the beauty in the middle, no matter how it looks on the surface.

We've spent the last few chapters talking about how we can change our thinking as we pursue deliberate movement, good nutrition, and a right attitude toward the scale. We want to set goals in those areas and move toward becoming the best and healthiest versions of ourselves. But in this chapter I want to help you understand that as you do that, your health journey will have a *middle* period—or likely more than one. There will be lulls, stops, sputters, failures, trials and retrials, and a myriad of other obstacles that separate where you are now from where you want to go. Sometimes when these challenges pop up, we give up and tell ourselves that we'll never reach our goals. But we don't have to settle for failure. I believe that the *middle* is one of the most formative spaces to solidify our plans for long-term health and wellness.

WHERE IS THE MIDDLE?

The middle is some *place* that is relevant to two points in a journey—a place between the beginning and the end, between north and south, or between life and death. Books and destinations have physical markers that are easy to place. If you find yourself lost on a drive between Miami and New York, you can whip out your GPS and plot your coordinates, quickly calculating the most efficient way to get to your final destination. Lose your place in a book? That's okay, just think back to the last thing you remember. You might have to flip a few pages, but you'll find it.

Health and fitness, however, don't have clear linear coordinates. Defining this journey as a point between two numbers on a scale is ill-advised because there will inevitably be all kinds of unexpected roadblocks and forward surges that cannot be precisely accounted for. If you're pursuing your best self the healthy way, you have to be somewhat flexible, willing to navigate an uncertain terrain when you're not sure what the end point is. So, the middle in this context is often just as difficult to find as a true beginning or end point. And unlike a linear story, the middle isn't only one place. You might find yourself in it often as your health and fitness change in conjunction with the pull of gravity or the number of times your body orbits around the sun.

I've told you about my defining beginning moment in this journey—the one where I cried all night, declaring that this time I was going to actually make the change. I see this moment as the start of my journey, even though so many aspects of my story began much earlier. But although my health journey has a beginning point, it doesn't yet have an end point. After reaching what I thought would be the stopping point multiple times, I've come to recognize that fitness, health, and being happy in my body are ever-moving goal posts. No matter what you achieve, you can always achieve more. So almost every part of the journey, then, is some sort of middle space. We are constantly between two coordinates, and it's a lot like driving in the mountains of Tennessee or Pennsylvania. Our journey is defined by highs and lows.

Seeing the beauty in both highs and lows will change your perspective. My husband grew up literally *on* a mountain. You could gaze out any window of the home he grew up in and see some sort of mountain chain. It was beautiful! He then moved to the Blue Ridge Mountains of Virginia for college (where we met) and basically traded one mountain chain

> Seeing the beauty in both highs and lows will change your perspective.

for another. It wasn't until life took us to Lawrence, Kansas, for him to get his doctorate degree that he realized the United States wasn't all beautiful mountains, hills, and valleys. If you pull up a map of the United States and zoom out, you can see that Lawrence, Kansas, is truly the "dead middle" of the country on a map. And, according to the American Geological Society, Lawrence is actually mathematically *flatter than a pancake*. On a clear day in Kansas on the highway, you can look ahead and see into a neighboring state, according to some truckers. We loved it there, and the scenery is as beautiful as the people. But it took a long time for us— particularly my mountain-born-and-raised husband—to appreciate it.

We now look back at that time and recognize that it was a middle period. We knew that we weren't going to be in Kansas forever (no one stays a student their entire life), but we also didn't know what was next. Would Phil get a job? Would we move? Where? We had general ideas about what was supposed to come next, but we also had to wrap our heads around the reality that we don't control every detail. At that point, it didn't seem like a middle because it was the present. It's only now that we've progressed past that point that we can frame it as such.

I think we need to reframe our health journeys in the same way. If you're reading this book, my guess is you have found yourself somewhere in the middle. The middle may vary from person to person because we all have different long- and short-term goals. You might be working toward a health goal like lower cholesterol or blood pressure, or a fitness goal like completing a 5K. You might want to feel more comfortable in your clothes. Or your goal might be something like nourishing your body in a way that makes you feel better. Whatever your goals, you're going to end up spending a lot of time in the middle. We all do. Because even when we meet one goal, we often set another—putting us squarely back in the middle again. So, to the fullest extent possible, enjoy that middle. It can be difficult to grapple with uncertainty and even frustrating to think about how to get to those end coordinates. But mountain highs are nothing without the valleys that help make them.

I invite you to settle in a bit. Enjoy your walk around the woods or the valley. Take in the scenery. Find solace and meaning in the middle, understanding that it is vitally important to your end coordinates. Let's talk about ways you can learn to appreciate your time in the middle, and perhaps even come to enjoy it, as you move forward in your journey.

REST

In the biblical account of creation, God works incredible wonders over the course of six busy days. Water and sky, grass and animals, humans sculpted from dust—he amazingly crafted the world like only he could ever do. But as fascinating as it is to ponder the mysteries of the creation of the world and all humanity, it's even more profound to consider what the most powerful being in all of time and space did on day seven.

He took a break.

God stepped back and saw that what he had made was good. He knew a messy situation was ahead, but for a moment his creation was good and complete, so he rested.

Of course we are not the same as God. Personally, I can't even make a good cake without following the instructions, so I know that sculpting humans out of dust isn't in my repertoire. Yet I find myself struggling with the honest truth that I often push myself beyond the measure that God originally intended. I *do, do, do, do, do* like a little baby shark, yet I never build in a moment to rest. If the God of the universe chose to take a time-out, I suspect that maybe it's good for our bodies to take one too.

I want to say this clearly: To overcome a stagnant season, you need rest. I see the need for rest manifest in two different ways. Most simplistically, our bodies need physical rest. I've talked to women who hustle in their diets and gym time. They take great pride in running themselves to the edge of exhaustion, as if it is a virtue to be upheld. It isn't. Fatigue is a real thing, and the body is an instrument. It was designed to carry out tasks, for sure, but it was also designed with a need for sleep, rest, and recovery. Just because your body *can* doesn't mean it *should*. If you've ever pulled an all-nighter to complete some task, you know this to be true. You can will your body to stay awake through the normal sleeping hours, but that obedience to your command comes with a price. Often that sleep cannot be fully recovered. You may actually weaken your immune system, limit your response times, and diminish your intellectual and cognitive capacities for meaningful human communication. We can't deny our bodies' need for physical rest.

But the second need for rest is much more along the lines of a *rest for the weary* motif. If you've birthed or adopted a child, you likely remember the first six months or so. Or maybe you don't. Sleepless nights, endless tears (yours and the baby's), 2 a.m. feedings. You didn't sleep. Thankfully, our children grow out of those moments as they become more independent. But what if they didn't? Can you even imagine? What if when you gave birth you were signing up for guaranteed sleepless nights for the next eighteen years? Let me temporarily take my "Mom of the Year" trophy off the shelf right now because if that were the case, I never would have signed up. We're able to get through those moments, though, because we realize they are temporary. They are fleeting. They won't last forever. If we can shift our thinking, we can actually come to enjoy the moments that wear us down because we realize they are equipping and building a future for the child we love beyond words. The moments are temporary, so the sacrifice is worth it.

Our health journey is more like this than not; our temporary sacrifices can build to a worthwhile long-term change. But so many of us have succumbed to the idea of a quick and easy fix—a fad diet here or a sadistic workout plan there. When these things don't work (and they never do), we feel once again that familiar sense of defeat, which quickly turns into self-doubt, which doesn't even bother to pause before whispering into our ears that we're going to be engaged in this battle for the rest of our lives. No. *This is a middle season.* It's the time where you are between big breakthroughs— between where you started and where you want to go. And it can feel like you'll be there forever.

But you won't.

You will get through this. But not without rest. First, physically rest your body. Second, rest in the journey. Lean into the reality that there is no quick fix and that there is no rapid blitz to some finish line (which will inevitably keep repositioning itself). Instead, choose to rest. Choose to be at peace with where you are right now in your health journey. Or, at the very least, choose to try to find it. That rest and that peace will help provide you with the clarity you need when it's time to move forward. If God, the creator of the universe, took the time for a breather before moving on to the next task, give yourself enough grace to do the same.

PATIENCE IS A VIRTUE

One reason I think we hate the middle is that we are profoundly impatient. Our lives are often chronicled by massive periods of waiting between significant life events.

You get engaged. Then you wait to walk down the aisle.

You get pregnant. Then you wait nine months to have the baby.

You get a job. Then you wait in longing for retirement.

Between moments that are worth chronicling, we often find ourselves waiting in the wings. As future-oriented thinkers, it is hard not to clamor for the next big fix. We're addicted to the feeling of accomplishing our next *next*. I believe in forward momentum and in setting goals we seek to accomplish. But I don't believe in the popular mantra that if you aren't moving forward, you're falling backward. I believe that sometimes the best way to clarify how to move forward is to pause, reflect, and consider before taking action.

There's a reason it's hard to wait for that moment where you walk down the aisle once you have the ring on your finger. It's easy to get lost in the excitement of it all—the details, the celebration, and the attention. But there's also a reason that most of us don't schedule the big day for the weekend after he gets down on one knee. Anything worth waiting for is worth the planning period it takes to complete it in excellence.

The same is true for our health journeys. We get lost in the *next*—the mental image we have of what it will be like when we reach whatever goal we're trying to reach. We think about what we'll be able to wear when we reach that size 14 or 8 or 2. We plan the celebration that will take place when we reach our goal and how we'll run to social media to share our update to the world. And whether we want to admit it or not, we often find ourselves obsessing about the attention that we'll receive once we lose weight—from our significant others, from our families, from those who counted us out, and from the general public.

Sure, there are outcomes and milestones we'll reach that can be celebrated and even propel us forward toward our next goal. But I want to invite you to accept the reality that patience leads to a more joyful journey. It is *good* to be patient. And if you want to feel *good*—in the gym, in your eating, in your view of yourself—take a look at how fixated you are on an end goal. Loosen your grip a little so you can appreciate where you are *right now*. Glance back to see how far you've come. Then turn your head forward with the right motive in mind. It's all intertwined. It's all important. And it's all part of what leads to a more enjoyable stroll toward feeling your best.

THE SCENIC ROUTE

Our lack of patience often centers on the fact that we are linear beings. Our entire physical existence is linear, marked with a clear beginning (our birth) and ending (our death). Yet as you've picked up on already, the real meat of the story comes from the stuff between those two defining moments. Linearity is a great tool because it hardwires us to be goal-oriented and equips us to keep reaching to be the best we can be—all worthwhile goals. But linear thinking can also limit us because it's the exact antithesis of stopping to smell the roses.

I'm going to pull on my firsthand experience here and tell you the truth. This journey is not linear. Even if you are the most dedicated, driven, strong-willed human being on the face of the planet, there are still some curvy roads you'll have to follow, some curveballs you'll have to watch for, and some curvy body characteristics you'll have to learn to embrace.

Maybe, just maybe, for this part of the road trip, you can take the scenic route, even if it doesn't race you to your destination on two wheels. You'll get to where you're going, but the journey will be much more enjoyable.

CURIOSITY KILLED THE CAT, BUT IT'LL MAKE A BETTER YOU

Our health pursuit is complex. It is so inherently personal, embedded with our own traumas (bullying), goals (not just a number on the scale!), histories (health profile), and more. When you find yourself in some sort of *middle*—whether that is a plateau or a need to put off to tomorrow what you simply can't do today—it is a good time to get curious with your own body.

We think of the human body and human experience as sort of "just there"—they are the mechanical interactions, movements, and moments that calculate to the sum of who we are. But we aren't robots. Each of us is designed for a specific purpose, and the corresponding DNA that houses that uniqueness courses through our life supply. If you've been on this health journey and are finding that things simply aren't working how you expected, maybe it's time that you get curious about the *hows* and *whys.*

This doesn't come naturally to me. Whereas my husband will question every aspect of a thing, always seeking to know the details, I'm a peacemaker at my core. I tend to accept things at face value. I don't go digging because I think we overcomplicate too much of life anyway. Why muddy the waters? But a few years ago, after my son was born, I went almost a year of not seeing a major budge in my progress (which was a main priority at the time). I grew impatient, frustrated, weary, and ultimately depressed. I succumbed to the weaknesses I tell others to watch out for—I got obsessive about the number on the scale. And after a full year, it finally dawned on me that I could turn my pity party into a much more fun party. I decided to get curious.

First, I consulted my doctor. I am a huge advocate of working with a medical professional on your health goals. My physicians have been infinitely kind and patient with me, despite my incessant (and often ridiculous) questions. But over the years, I've developed a relationship with them and feel comfortable baring my heart and soul. So, when I reached my plateau and brought them some of my familiar elixir of despair, they listened and offered to do some blood tests that might reveal any hormone imbalances or other conditions that could be affecting my health and slowing my metabolism. I was so excited . . . and then disappointed. Because, true to all that I preach, I discovered there was no easy fix. I was fine. My blood, to put it in medical terminology, was *totes fine*. There was no pill that could fix me and no diagnosis that could explain me.

Okay . . . onto the next thing. I took a careful inventory of my eating. I tried going gluten free. I tried keto. I tried the bread diet (just kidding—that's not a thing, but if it was, I'd be on that). I tried vegetarianism, veganism, and a myriad of eating styles (note: not crash diets, which are generally geared toward restricting calories; by that point, I had learned my lesson) to see if it shifted my plateau. But food wasn't the easy fix I was looking for.

Fine. I'm resilient. I knew I'd find out what was holding back my progress. Next, I adjusted my workout style. I felt like I was already going pretty hard, but I was sure that I'd find it within me to go harder. I tried. I really did. I bumped my workout schedule from four days a week to six or sometimes even seven. I ramped up my lifting, ran faster, trained harder. But as much as I increased my efforts, things were still not changing. Until they changed for the worse. I started working out like a crazy woman, stopping at nothing to rid my arms of the extra fluff that plagued them, and then *crack*—my shoulder offered a rebuttal. So I found myself back chatting with my doctor, this time sore in both my arm and my soul. Another thing that didn't work.

Ever patient, that doctor watched me wipe the running mascara from my face and let me have my mini-meltdown. Then she finally told me the words I had been dying to hear: "I think I know what's wrong with you." The tears stopped flowing immediately and the corners of my mouth started to turn up. *I knew it! Finally, I was going to get my answer.* She paused before spilling the (disappointing) beans: "You're a mom. You're working full-time. Life is busy. It's exhausting. You, Jennifer . . . are *tired*!" I waited for the "Aha! Gotcha!" to follow, but there wasn't one. She was serious. After letting the pause linger just a bit, she let me down gently, noting that she commonly sees moms of young children struggling to balance it all. In fact, she let me know that I wasn't alone. I wasn't the only one who wondered *What's wrong with me?* because I was stuck in the middle between my health goals. I was busy, life was crazy and exhausting, and I was a woman trying hard to balance the chaos the best I could from day to day.

Though this wasn't the answer I was hoping for, I could finally lean into the reality that sometimes I couldn't balance it all. And I could also lean into the feeling of satisfaction. Rather than negatively framing my endless pursuit for answers as being all for naught, I saw it as a moment of understanding. I wasn't some crazy woman. I was a woman on a mission, and I'd used all the resources I had to make sense of my situation. I got curious about every aspect of my health and, though none of those curiosities gave me *the* answer, they gave me many answers. I discovered parts of my health that had actually improved since my unhealthy early adult years (thanks, blood panel!). Through looking at nutrition, I discovered the foods that sit well with me and those that don't (dairy and I are like colleagues that get along, but we definitely aren't besties). And I discovered that hard workouts are good, but too much does more to exacerbate my situation than it does to help it.

In my season of curiosity, I learned a lot about myself. To me, that's a great way to grapple with the reality of being in the middle. Now I know more about who I am, what works, what doesn't, and why.

While you're on the scenic route, take some time to get curious about your own body. Take notice of what change your body might be asking you for. Just because there's a low-carb craze running wild out there doesn't mean *your* body isn't begging you for some carbs. Just because running has always been your go-to exercise doesn't mean that's the one your body loves the most. Or maybe it does! Only you know. Get curious about what your body wants and needs and be free to explore those things.

GRAPPLE WITH FAILURE

I couldn't wait to get my license. The moment I turned sixteen, I begged my mom to take me to the DMV for my test. And once I passed, I couldn't wait to get my hands on the decade-old steering wheel of my first car—a rusty white Firebird. I drove that thing around endlessly, and it lasted a good while until it did what most cheap cars do—it started to nickel-and-dime me. I found myself on the side of the busy highway in my Florida town more times than I'd like to remember.

When I was old enough to move on to a more mature car, I slid into the seat of my second car, a base-level Dodge Neon. This one was also white but without the rust. I thought I could rest assured that it would run smoothly and that my days on the side of the road were over—but I was wrong. I remember when my husband was only my boyfriend and I'd have to call him to come pick me up in our little college town to get to class, church, or the grocery store because that Neon had one fun trick: It liked to throw its transmission. I pumped thousands of dollars into that car over my years as a college student whose money wasn't exactly free-flowing.

I kept trying to keep it alive, but by the time I replaced the transmission for the third time, I decided I wasn't putting one more cent into that thing.

In the early years of our relationship, my husband and I bought older cars and ended up with lots of breakdowns. Fed up with buying cars, we finally paused, looked at each other, and thought, *We must be approaching this whole car-buying thing completely wrong.* We shifted mindsets and decided we'd be better off purchasing a newer car, in better shape, with a still-active warranty so that maybe we'd finally rid ourselves of nonstop car problems. Five years later, here we are—still driving that car that has caused no stress at all.

And boy, do I appreciate the trusty Toyota Highlander that totes my littles around every day without any problems. This car is meaningful to me. We had to sacrifice to get it at the time, but that sacrifice meant something to us because we understand what it's like to have cars that fail. We understand what it's like to be left on the side of the road, having to call a tow truck and figure out how to pay for major car repairs. The reality we have now has been made so much sweeter by the failure and sacrifice we've had to endure.

The same can be true with our health journeys. Failure (perhaps more easily digestible when we call it "trial and error") has a way of making the realities of our situation crystal clear. I've certainly failed many times in my journey. I've done too little and let my body get to an unhealthy state. I've done too much and required extensive healing to bring my body back to its normal state. I've regressed after making progress because I've had to tend to other things. But each of those failures taught me valuable life lessons. Failure doesn't have to be negative. Though it often feels insurmountable, failure—for most of us—is never permanent.

I believe we can reframe failure as a rest stop. If you found out you were lost on a highway or driving the wrong direction on a trip to New York from Miami, you wouldn't keep going, would you? No way! You'd recognize that you were wasting valuable time that could be spent shopping in Soho or eating decadent food in Midtown. But you'd also know that without stopping to take a look at where you were and how to reroute, you'd be foolish for just cranking a U-turn and going the other way. When you recognize that you've failed—in whatever capacity that may be—don't succumb to the pressure to right that wrong without even pausing to consider the road ahead. See failure as a place where you can pull over, reframe, and calculate the best path forward. Don't berate yourself for not reaching your goals.

A quote often attributed to Winston Churchill defines success as stumbling from failure to failure with no loss of enthusiasm. I'd invite you to do just this when you recognize that you've "failed" and found yourself stuck in the middle as a result. Be honest with where you stand and what that means for where you're going. But use that rest stop to calibrate your perspective, seeing failure as an

> See failure as a place where you can pull over, reframe, and calculate the best path forward.

opportunity to further test what works and what doesn't. It's easy to hastily define "the middle" as a space entirely categorized by failure, but don't. Instead, see it as a space where you can learn what failure, and ultimately, what *success*, even means.

YOU'RE FINDING YOURSELF

The middle isn't always the most fun part of our journey. Just ask Cinderella. No one wants to find themselves confused about what lies ahead, frustrated that it hasn't arrived yet, and toiling in the dark trying to achieve it. But stories—yours included—have a middle for a reason. These ebbs and flows (or hills and valleys) in our life's narrative give us character. They give us purpose. They build resilience. They often confuse and clarify at the same time. That's their function. The purpose of the middle is to provide context. A difficult middle makes a rewarding ending all the more worth it. We can celebrate our accomplishments in health and fitness so much more when we step back and recognize the middle gives us the *real* story—the sleepless nights, the discomfort and failure that ultimately lead to more determination, more focused work, and more success.

I hope that you won't diminish the middle. I love the Arabian proverb that reminds us, "All sunshine and no rain makes a desert." Learn to enjoy the little storms that life affords in your fitness journey, and see what you can learn from them. I think this anonymous author got it right:

"Sometimes you find yourself in the middle of nowhere, and sometimes in the middle of nowhere, you find yourself."

Flip the Script

Instead of telling yourself, "I can never seem to reach my goals," say this instead: **"I am thankful for my journey and excited to see where it takes me."**

Reflect

As you look back on your life, where have you felt stuck in the middle? What are some things you have learned from your time in the middle? How can you begin to appreciate the middle and lean into the benefits of actually enjoying it?

Action Step

Swap your normal route for a scenic route to work or school (or wherever you normally go), and look for the beauty in it. Imagine how much better your health journey would be if you learned to do the same.

Chapter 10

LOVE THE SKIN YOU'RE IN

The nurse smiles and pulls the curtain closed as she backs out of the room, leaving me with a paper gown to slip into. I smile back; this is the day I've been waiting for. My thumbs gently remove the pajama pants they told me to wear this morning, and I throw them to the side. I'm shedding so much today. My fingers pull apart my cotton-knit top, each button another step toward parting ways with what I've been chained to for years.

My eyes catch a glimpse of my body in the full-length mirror across the room. I wonder how many women have allowed their inner critics to run wild while they're looking into that mirror; how many have made life-changing decisions based on the girl staring back at them; how many think that this huge step in the journey will finally bring them what they've been searching for.

I pull on the paper gown, leaving it open in the front. No sooner do I climb onto the table than the nurse comes back into the room, this time with a needle. She sticks me a few times, since my veins are being finicky this morning. Finally, she gets one. This is it.

A few minutes later my husband walks into the room. I smile and give him a kiss. Only nine hours until I'll see his sweet face again. I'll be loopy and the drugs won't have worn off quite yet, but at least by then he'll know I've made it through. His eyebrows look droopy. He forces a smile, but I can see the fear in his eyes. He warns that I better wake up from the anesthesia. He reminds me six times how much he loves me. I already know that to be true. He'd love me if I didn't go through with this. If I stayed this way forever. He has always made me feel like the most beautiful woman he's ever seen.

But still, I'm determined.

As they lift the bed's brakes and start wheeling me back, I reminisce about how long I've awaited this moment. I daydream about how different things will be.

We enter the big, sterile room. There's no going back. The lights are beaming down, peering into every detail they touch. The bed is still now. We must be waiting for the nurses to get everything into place—the scalpels and other tools suitable for cutting away that which is no longer welcome. I look around the room. I didn't realize it took so many people to make this happen. What are they all working on as they scurry around the room in their cobalt scrubs? Each seems so intent on their task. I make some small talk. I smile, nervously hoping they all got a good night of rest and that I wake up when this is all said and done.

They hook me up to the anesthesia, and all the nerves drift away as I fall into a deep sleep.

Today is the day I trade my skin for scars.

SKIN BY THE HANDFULS

What people don't always realize about massive weight loss is the aftermath. You work your butt off (literally) to lose the weight and you're left with handfuls of loose skin that won't go away with any amount of water, vitamins, exercise, or perfect nutritional habits. Trust me, I've tried them all.

The only way to get the bulk of the loose skin to go away is through surgery. And this is not a fun, quick office visit covered under a co-pay. We're talking a *head to a plastic surgeon, save all your dollars and pay out of pocket, spend eight weeks recovering from the massive physical journey your body just underwent* type of ordeal.

I am lined with scars now, and I haven't forgotten how desperately I wanted these incision marks in return for the loose skin that embellished my body. When my second-born was merely months old, I was already scheduling consultations with surgeons so I could discuss my options. Three separate surgeons took a look at my unclothed body and assessed what it would take to rid me of the burden I was carrying. It would require several surgeries, and even then all the extra skin might not be gone. But in my mind, it was worth it.

The loose skin was a mark of a tremendous accomplishment. After all, losing 160 pounds was no easy trek. It took years, and a complete shift in my lifestyle and habits. On the one hand, I was proud to be draped in loose skin because it meant that the fat had escaped. That's what happens: Your skin expands to accommodate being so large, but it loses elasticity and doesn't tighten back into place when you shrink back down. My loose skin was a remnant of my story.

Yet my pride in what I'd accomplished didn't negate how uncomfortable it was to carry this baggage. I'd tuck it all into some high-waisted compression pants during workouts, but still the skin would tug at my lower back during push-ups or burpees. Without the compression pants I could get into a plank position, and while my back and legs would be a straight line, my tummy would sweep the surface of the floor. It wasn't filled with fat. It was just that my skin was *that* loose.

When you're fat, at least your skin is tight—it holds you in. When you lose the weight and the skin that once held that fat in becomes saggy, it causes uncomfortable shifting inside your body. Your organs aren't tightly held and it hurts. Even going for a run has its challenges. When I ran, with every touch of my foot to the pavement, gravity would pull my belly apron down, yanking all the way to my lower back. By the end of it I was walking hunched over.

After years of dealing with it, I decided I'd rather live with the scars than the skin. Yet the decision to move forward with surgery didn't mean I could just run out the door and climb onto an operating table. It would be years before I was actually able to have the procedure. We'd have to save up tens of thousands of dollars to make it happen. We'd have to find room on the calendar for Phil to be on kid-duty for an extended period of time. We'd have to make sure I wouldn't birth any more children, at least for a few years.

Day after day I'd tuck the loose skin into my clothing, hoping no one would notice it. I'd strip off my clothes to climb into the shower and I'd peer in the mirror in anguish over it. People would say, "But isn't it better than carrying the fat?" and I'd of course agree. But they didn't understand just how exasperating it was. And they wouldn't. After a while you get tired of explaining your loose skin problem over and over again to skinny people who think you're talking about getting liposuction. So you smile and nod.

And why is fat so much worse than the skin anyway? What makes fat so terrible, awful, and uncomfortable for so many people?

I wondered that as a child. When kids would make fun of me in school, I remember crying to my mom, asking her why people hated my fat so much. It wasn't like the fat was on *their* bodies. It didn't cause them pain or interfere with their lives in any way. They could easily just look away if they didn't want to see it. But there was some reason unbeknownst to me that fat was repulsive to people—so much that they would literally spew words of hatred toward me. To this day I don't understand why people have such a problem with that three-letter word.

I used to think I was the only one who dealt with excess skin from weight loss, but in recent years I've seen plenty of people on Instagram and in real life share their skin struggles. It's a common issue among those of us who have lost upward of 100 pounds. Knowing that I'm not alone softened the sting of what was lingering under my clothes.

At first I was sad that I couldn't rush right out and get the surgery, but now I'm glad I had to wait a while. The delay caused me to process so many deeper elements of my understanding of total health and wellness.

NOT RIGHT NOW

I'll never forget driving home from one of our initial consultations when the reality hit. My ever-supportive husband looked at me and said, "Babe, I love you and I'll do anything for you, but you know we don't have the money for this surgery yet, right?"

"I know," I replied, forcing a smile.

I looked out the window and the all-too-familiar tears started streaming down my face. What was I thinking even scheduling the consultation? I knew there was no way we could afford to get even one phase of the surgery right now. And the fact that it would take several surgeries meant that the price tag, when all was said and done, would mirror a person's annual salary. Or more, even. Why did I get my hopes up? How could I possibly spend years in this body draped in skin? When would the day actually come? What if we were *never* able to make it happen?

That moment was a major turning point in my journey toward self-love. Because when the tears dried up, I had a decision to make. Either I could hate every second of living in this skin-excessive body, or I could learn to have a healthier perspective. I decided right then that I would trust God to help us make the surgery happen when he deemed it was the right timing and that I would start working on my body perception in the meantime.

> When the tears dried up, I had a decision to make. Either I could hate every second of living in this skin-excessive body, or I could learn to have a healthier perspective.

Most people think that when you get skin surgery you're doing it only because you want to look better. When I eventually got my surgery, so many people asked me if I finally felt like a million bucks when I went to the beach or if I liked my new tummy. Those questions, while well-intended, made me cringe a little. Because in my heart of hearts I knew that my appearance was not my primary motive for getting the surgery. Don't get me wrong, I do like my tummy, and I do feel more comfortable heading to the beach. But it's not because I traded in my rags for rock-hard abs. It's because I had to fight tooth-and-nail to love my body in the in-between time.

The years between losing the weight and losing the skin were formative for me. I pursued health and wellness intently, improving my fitness, developing a better relationship with food, and most of all, learning to accept who I was where I was. So no—I didn't feel like a million bucks after losing the skin; I felt like a million bucks when I went to the gym with it tucked in my pants and still did all the moves. I felt like a million bucks when I finally shed the weight *and* the idea that I didn't need to let my body define my entire life journey. The skin removal process made me look more like the aesthetic standard that people expected of me post-weight loss, but it didn't change me the way fighting through my body image issues did.

HOW TO GET A BIKINI BODY

One of my biggest passions is body positivity—but let me be clear that I didn't just start preaching that message only after I had the skin removed. Though it was uncomfortable at times, I learned to live at peace with my extra skin. Gradually, during those post-weight-loss, loose-skin years, I ramped up my courage to live my life without fear of what others thought about my body.

I'll never forget when I marched right into my favorite clothing store with one specific goal in mind: to buy a bikini. My first one ever. I was coming to terms with the fact that I'd be living with saggy skin, and I wanted to pursue true peace with the body I was living in. With butterflies in my stomach, I headed to the swimsuit section and grabbed a high-waisted bottom and a floral-patterned top. Our family would be heading to the beach in a couple of days, and I was going to push past my comfort zone and dive into the confidence club. Loose skin and all.

Beach day arrived and I excitedly threw on my new wardrobe piece. I looked in the mirror and butterflies filled my whole body. Thoughts of loathing filled my head. *Are you really going to do this? Look at your saggy skin. Look at how big your legs are. Your tan is uneven. Your back rolls are showing. You bought the wrong kind of top. There's a perfectly good one-piece in the top drawer of the dresser. Go grab that instead.*

I shut up the critical voice and reminded myself that it didn't matter what anyone at the beach thought—I was there for me, not them. I rounded up the kids and hubby and we headed out. I prepped myself the whole way for the judgmental stares and even perhaps a comment or a snicker I was going to get from others. I was ready, and I knew that what was inside me was worth far more than my external appearance.

We got to the beach, we parked, and we walked. And then, guess what happened? Absolutely nothing. No odd looks by fellow beachgoers. No bullies spewing words at me like when I was a child. My kids didn't think anything of it. No one did—except my husband, who knows me at my core and grinned from ear to ear when he saw his wife walk right onto that powdery sand with confidence (he's a *good* man, but he's still a man).

No one was hating my body. When would I get that through my head? People aren't sitting around critiquing our bodies. I mean, sure, there are a few bad apples out there.

But most people aren't running rampant with their hateful thoughts about our muffin tops or the cellulite on our bums. And guaranteed: If they are, it's likely because they're super hard on themselves, and their own inner critic is so strong that it leaks out toward others.

Confidence outranks perfection any day.

I learned in that moment that confidence outranks perfection any day. And I had many more opportunities to practice that confidence. Our family was living in Florida at the time, just a short drive away from two of the most beautiful beaches in the country. And each time we visited, I'd throw on that two-piece swimsuit and will myself to muster up confidence. It felt odd at first, but I was determined to get over this hurdle.

Slowly the walls around my heart started to fall. And as they did, I was able to see the world around me more clearly. I realized that I was dumping all of my energy into anxiety-ridden thoughts of insecurity, while other people were soaking up the sunshine, building sandcastles with their kids, and floating their worries away in the waves of the ocean.

I wanted to be like that. I wanted to go to the beach and forget to worry about what I looked like in a swimsuit. I wanted to laugh and smile with my littles and have my joy be real. I wanted to sit in the sand and not be consumed with the way my belly fluff was folding onto itself.

I wanted that *more* than I wanted to sit on the beach with the perfect body.

It was four years between that first day and the day we took our last trip to that breathtaking beach before moving out of state. Within those four years I completely rewrote the dialogue inside my head that narrates how I view my body. It's a combination of loving my body and simply not letting my body (in whatever shape it is at any given moment) take up so much of my headspace. During that last trip to the beach I didn't think about how I looked. Instead, my eyes scanned the horizon of the ocean as the sun set. I felt the breeze in my hair. I stretched my arms around my husband's shoulders, kissed him, and looked into the depth of his beautiful blue eyes. I watched my babies chase seagulls, splash water, and collect seashells. I thanked God for giving us a handful of years in the Sunshine State, and I eagerly anticipated the new season of life that awaited our family.

TO THOSE WHO WAIT

While I was working on loving my body as is, we were also saving up money for the skin surgery and working toward setting aside a chunk of time in which I would be able to focus on the eight-week recovery period that comes along with such a hefty procedure. A couple of years passed after that initial consultation, our son was getting a little older, we were finally feeling rooted living in Florida, and we felt it was time to venture into surgery land. We'd take it one surgery at a time, starting with what's called a 360-degree lower body lift. This meant I'd have an incision around the entire circumference of my abdomen and lower back. Phil about fainted handing over the check at the surgeon's office; yet we both knew it was worth it since we'd both carried the uncomfortable excess skin that comes with significant weight loss. We set the appointment for just a few days after my thirty-fourth birthday, and I started counting down the weeks and days.

I had waited so long for this surgery, and I knew for certain that I wanted to have it done. No second-guessing on my end. A friend of mine who had had a similar surgery gave me some words of advice: "It's not an easy recovery, Jennifer. Just make sure you're *sure* you want to do it."

I was sure.

When I lay down on the bed before going into the operating room, I reshuffled my abdominal skin *overflow* underneath my gown, as if even in that last final moment, I felt a duty to make sure my body looked as acceptable as possible as the nurses peeled back my clothes in the surgical suite. As they had me count backward from ten before the anesthesia kicked in, I couldn't help but have one of those *life flashing before my eyes* moments. I was happy, of course; but I was also angry. Here I was, about to be cut open in a multihour surgery that, though safe, came with risks—all because this body had demanded so much of me. I pushed those thoughts aside, quickly replacing them with a prayer and gratitude before closing my eyes and settling into deep sleep that this mama of two hadn't known for nearly a decade.

I did, however, wake up much like I do on any given Saturday to the sound of kids ~~playing peacefully~~

fighting—groggy. I felt so many emotions but nothing physically. I was numb. I couldn't believe the skin was gone! Yet I felt not even one degree different than I had before the procedure. I guess I had thought that, though they wheeled my Cabbage Patch body to the operating room, they'd bring me back looking like Barbie. Didn't happen.

My friend was right—recovery was no joke. I dozed in and out of consciousness, chomping ice chips and devouring whatever home renovation show was on TV. When the nurse came into the room at 5:30 the next morning, it was time to get on my feet for the first time post-surgery. I thought it would be easy, but it wasn't. It felt like my abdomen was loaded with bricks; I couldn't stand up even partially straight. I had this odd thought that my incision might burst open with all the pressure, even though the nurse had assured me it wouldn't. I slowly inched my way into the bathroom and sat on the toilet seat while the nurse scurried around preparing for our next big first. The surgeon had put four drains into my lower abdomen area to get rid of built-up fluid that accumulates post-surgery, and it was time to empty my drains for the first time. As the nurse started with drain one, I became light-headed and nauseous. With the drip, drip, drips of the drains came also the drip, drip, drips from my eyes.

I felt a rush of emotions. As much as those tears were a reflection of the pain I felt physically in that moment, so, too, were they a salty reminder of the battle I'd had with myself over the past thirty-odd years—a battle that played out on my physical body. Though I'd presumed the surgery would end the battle, in that moment I realized I was actually in the middle of it.

THE VALUE OF WAITING

I'm glad I had to wait a long time before I got the surgery. And I'm not just saying that because that's how people soothe the frustration of not getting what they want when they want it. The waiting period was valuable in the long run because it prepared my heart and mind to believe my body was good. Because after the newness of the surgery wore off and the pain and swelling subsided, I looked in the mirror, and guess what I saw?

Imperfections.

The lower-body lift targeted only the skin on my abdominal and lower back area. Loose skin still covered just about everywhere else on my body. Subsequent surgeries would help with that, but that was still down the road a bit.

Now I saw scars that would never go away.

Arms that were still covered in loose skin and thighs that were just the same.

Wait a minute. The surgery took away your extra skin but didn't take away the negative thoughts you had about yourself? Honestly? Nope. I still saw all the things I deemed flaws. That body anxiety we feel is an inherently emotional and biological response. Sometimes I wonder if many of us get a rush of dopamine when we belittle our bodies because we've come to see restrictive eating or self-deprecation as a rite of passage instead of a perverse misunderstanding of what it means to be human.

Though I had melted the fat off of my body through years of hard work and then *cut off* ten pounds of the human body's largest organ through this skin removal surgery—I recognized that unless I cut away part of my brain too, the operation would be for naught. The waiting process helped me pre-negotiate some of my post-surgery feelings. Although some of that body anxiety still emerged as a temptation, that wait gave me the necessary space I needed to squash it as it arose.

In that in-between time before the surgery, I dedicated space to pray, reflect, and plan for the changes and recovery my body would undergo. That might sound extreme, but the depth of my body trauma is significant to me, and it emerges as a disruption to so many other elements of my life—my family, my professional career, the risks I take, the activities I engage in, and the company I keep. I knew that pause was important because it allowed me to sit with the fact that no amount of external changes to my body would automatically make me love what I saw in the mirror.

I had to realize that surgery doesn't leave you with the perfect anything—a point solidified after I healed. Yes, my tummy is bit flatter now, but I still have quite a bit of loose skin. All the stretch marks are still there. I still have love handles. With all of the wonder of his skilled hands, my surgeon didn't and couldn't just magically tighten every fiber of my skin. I've had two additional surgeries since then, and as I type these words I still have one more major surgery that

I'll undergo when I feel ready. My legs are still swimming in loose skin, and I have scars that extend from my elbow to my armpit and all the way down my sides. People see those scars all the time, perhaps noticing them even more than I thought they were noticing my overweight or over-skinned body.

But even I am surprised at how I feel about those scars, which could easily be seen as horrific reflections of a lifetime of body and weight issues. I don't cringe when my eyes gravitate toward scars or skin on this good body of mine. I don't regret my decision for surgery in any way; in fact, I see it as just another chapter in this very long trek. Another hard hurdle that I jumped over. More than forty inches of faded incision lines remind me of how far I have come in this thing we call a health journey. Decade-old stretch marks stare at me with intent, and I smile with compassion and gratitude. I'm not intimidated by these off-kilter body embellishments; I'm inspired by them.

It's important to realize that many of our battles with our bodies are not really about the body at all—they are about the mind. We think we can learn to be content the way we are. Then we think that we might be *more* content if we dropped the weight. Then we think that we might be *even more* content if we got the skin removed (or had some other form of cosmetic intervention). None of those things are inherently bad! But as someone who has been through those self-defeating thought cycles, I have learned that none offer true freedom.

And when you realize that, it becomes quite easy to enter into another defeating cycle of negative self-talk, where guilt and condemnation come in. I've had that, too.

You say you're "body positive" but you've had plastic surgery?

You say that you don't need to be skinny to be sexy but you still wear Spanx?

You say to love your body as is, but you still have to work at it some days.

POSITIVE ABOUT MY CHANGING BODY

I want to be clear in this chapter: Loving your body doesn't mean that you can't pursue better health, or skin removal surgery, or a new hair color, or whatever else. I've never regretted my surgeries; I'm glad I had each one of them. But it was important that I did them for me, not to try to appease society, fix my body-image issues, or try to fit some unrealistic ideal. I'm not the one to dictate what you should or should not pursue in terms of living your healthiest life. Only you can decide that. It's not about putting yourself in a box and never changing. It's about viewing your body through the right lens. It's about carrying peace and confidence in who you are and not allowing your critical thoughts to drive you into unhealthy patterns or behaviors.

I want us all to step back and recognize that a motivation to change can be healthy if tailored correctly. But it's that *tailoring* that we need to calibrate. We need to check our motive.

Not every decision I've made has been driven by the right

motive. I'm quite sure that that crash diet I mentioned in an earlier chapter was not driven by a desire to have healthy habits and an overall balanced lifestyle. Nope, it was probably just to lose weight. And my first skin removal consult—many, many years ago and well before I got the surgery—wasn't nearly as self-love-motivated as the one I got years later when I actually moved forward because I felt ready to do it in a healthy way.

Motive matters. It matters in weight loss, in exercise, when you're donning a swimsuit for the beach, and yes, it matters in cosmetic surgery. In every single leg (and arm and thigh) of my journey, I have had to learn this lesson. It doesn't come naturally for me—I have to work at it. Subconsciously, *I* get that dopamine rush when I think negatively about my body. Deep down within me, I feel as if it is only normal to identify and reflect on my imperfections. That's deep, and it comes from multiple places of trauma. But trauma can cripple us or it can inform our approach as we move forward, and that's what I'm willing it to do for me. I recognize on an even deeper spiritual level that there is purpose in my (past) pain and that with the right motive, that story of pain and purpose can inspire others to be free from the prison of body anxiety.

When you're not just seeking skinny or wallowing in self-loathing, when you're committed to loving yourself, when you see your body as good and want to treat it with respect by becoming the best and healthiest version of yourself, you can begin to write a new story that builds on your past. With the right motive, your pain can all be made *worth it.*

It's worth it to me as I sit here in my size _____ jeans and my size _____ shirt, not caring about that actual size and what it might be next month, next year, or in the next decade. It's worth it when I get on the scale after a vacation and it says I'm "up" five pounds, but I'm *not* filled with fear that I'm heading back to a place of utter body defeat and failure. It's worth it when I go out to dinner with my family and treat myself to a yummy meal that I'm not guilt-ridden about. It's worth it when I see my daughter talk about bodies having fat or "fluffiness" and seeing that she has no negative understanding of perfectly human attributes. It's worth it when my husband spontaneously grabs my love handles and instead of being embarrassed I'm ready to run up to the bedroom with him. It's worth it when I walk into a room and don't wonder who thinks I'm fatter than they are. It's worth it, my friend, to check your motive because I believe most of our body issues come from misplaced motives.

It's worth the effort it takes to change your thinking patterns about yourself. It's worth it to see yourself the way God sees you. Because, newsflash—you are loved *deeply* with fat, with extra skin, with wrinkles, and even with that chin beard you try to wax away. You're more than welcome to address any places on your body that you'd like; just remember to do it with the right motive.

Plastic surgery won't fix your body issues.

Nor will a crash diet.

Nor the best chin-beard waxer in the world.

But if you can fix your motive—if you can learn to pursue changes because you want what is best for yourself and not because you feel unworthy unless you improve—you can alleviate many of your body issues, even as you work to customize the template of your body as you see fit. Whatever you decide, be sure you're doing it *for you*.

Flip the Script

Instead of telling yourself, "I'll be happy if I just . . . ," say this instead: **"I can be happy with myself right now, as I am today."**

Reflect

What would it take to look at yourself in the mirror with love instead of disgust? How could you change the lens through which you see yourself?

Action Step

Buy a two-piece swimsuit or another article of clothing you don't usually wear because you're afraid of others' opinions. Remember you're just as worthy to wear it as anyone else, and you're doing it for you.

Chapter 11

LOVE YOUR BODY
(EVEN WHEN YOU DON'T)

When I was in middle school I took a trip to Toronto with my dad. It was truly magical; even in my teenage angst, I was able to find deep appreciation for how much effort he put into making that trip special. And on our last evening there, we found ourselves eating dinner at a restaurant with one of the most beautiful views I've ever seen. Between the main course and dessert, we left the table and walked over to the sky view area to take it all in. I must have looked dumbstruck staring out the window toward the city skyline. "Don't you just wish you could stay here forever?" my dad asked sweetly. "Yeah," I said with a dreamy sigh—utterly in awe of the landscape. Yet the sweetness of the moment was a little lost when, without skipping a beat, he said, "Well, you can't," laughed a little, and walked back to our table.

Talk about rushing straight back to reality. But perhaps he had it right all along. You can't stay here forever.

I'm not talking about Toronto. I'm talking about this space that you—that *we*—all want to be: somewhere we're healthy in every way. But too often we can't stay here because our ideas about our bodies keep us from being fully healthy.

Tons of women come to me, year after year, asking for help with weight loss. And while in recent years I've shifted away from coaching weight loss and focused more on food freedom, I *do* have answers for them. I have helped many people adopt a healthier lifestyle and redefine their view of themselves along the way. I *do* understand what it takes to adopt a mindset shift in this area of life. But the truth is, I still feel inadequate to share these healthy lifestyle tweaks with others at times.

Why? Because *I* don't have the ideal body we see dancing around on social media and on magazine covers.

Try as I might to bump these notions from my head, I often feel pressed to really buckle down and lose more weight, or lean out, or bulk up, or . . .

I remember sitting at breakfast with some new friends and chatting about our lives as young moms struggling to make it in the complicated world we live in. Since we were getting to know one another, I was—in true Jennifer form—*word vomiting* my whole story out onto the table for them. (It's truly a weakness, y'all.) I told them about my weight-loss journey, how I started focusing on body positivity, and beyond. At one point I mentioned the many women who message me asking for help with losing weight. I remember feeling a little embarrassed as I shared with my new friends that I felt like an imposter in those conversations. I figured they could easily understand why I would feel weird offering others any words of wisdom on this topic. After all, they could both see that I'm not the size and frame of most women you see empowering others to become their healthiest selves. But to my surprise, one of them asked for clarification.

"I'm sorry, I don't understand. Why do you feel inadequate to offer help to those who are seeking a healthier lifestyle?"

Wait. Did she not notice the elephant in the room?

Like, me. I'm the elephant. You know? Jennifer with the big arms, big thighs, Cabbage Patch–doll cheeks?

I sort of chuckled it off and skirted around the answer, and the conversation moved on. But on my drive home, I replayed her question over and over again in my mind. How could she not tell that the reason I feel weird offering weight-loss advice is because I don't have a body that others want? I thought about my outfit choice for that morning; maybe my clothes were more figure-flattering than I realized. Maybe I somehow looked a little smaller that day than I thought. Maybe it was the way I was sitting; perhaps the table was covering my muffin top and she couldn't see what was hiding there. Maybe the darker color of my jacket made me look thinner.

If she'd seen me clearly, I was sure she would have understood my question: Who would want to take body advice from a girl who looks like me?

That's the pendulum in my mind, ever swinging back and forth. Sometimes I say to myself, "*Girl*! You did that thing! Look at how far you've come in your health journey! Now go help others!"

And other times I think there's no way in this world someone would want to hear health tips from someone in a body like mine. They want to hear from the health coach who's got ripped abs, 4 percent body fat, and only drinks double-pressed vegan honeybee pollen smoothies for breakfast.

That's not me—and it never will be.

I think I've finally—maybe—gotten to the place where I realize that perhaps being me, just as I am, is my calling. It's a part of my purpose. I think about another meal I shared with a pastor friend of mine who was hoping I would agree to lead a women's wellness group at her church. We spent some time eating good food and getting to know each other. Then she dived right into why she wanted me to help the women in her church adopt healthier habits. At first I sat there surprised that she would ask *me* when there are so many other more fitting women to lead such a group. But I'll never forget what she told me.

She said, "Jennifer, I see so many fitness experts out there helping other women, but I cannot bring myself to follow the advice of someone who already looks like a body builder. I can't relate to that. You, on the other hand, have massive success in the area of healthy living, but you seem like a *real* person. You're not consumed with being perfect in your eating, exercise, and perception of yourself. You're just a normal person who is always striving toward your healthiest self. That's why I learn from you, and that's why I want you to pour into the women at my church."

It was as if God spoke directly through her, giving me confirmation that it was okay for me to be *me* and that *I* was enough. I needed those words and I still cling to those words. Let's be honest; many of us are more fragile than we care to admit. Often, our deepest insecurities are the hardest ones to overwrite. But in our vulnerability, our greatest purpose can really shine.

While writing this book, I was struck by the startling revelation that I've spent more of my days loathing my body than I have appreciating and loving it. We all have our own experiences and our own pain. But this is the chapter where we turn away from that weeping. It's about not letting defeat shape the way we see ourselves but beginning to see ourselves as we truly are. The way God sees us.

F.A.T.

When my daughter was in first grade, one of the smaller girls in her class just so happened to talk about fat out loud on the playground one day. From there, she began to sort her classmates by their sizes. "You're not really fat *or* skinny, Kennedy," she said. My blood boiled when my daughter recounted this, but Kennedy seemed largely unbothered.

I pressed a bit more, but when she didn't divulge I settled on a little ditty: "None of us *is* fat. We just *have* fat." She seemed satisfied.

I went about my day after dropping her off in the school car line, but I kept thinking about that sticky statement. It had flown out of my mouth quickly in an attempt to smooth over any concerns she might have about her size as a mere six-year-old. But as I began to reflect on the value of self-love and reframing the way we see ourselves, I looked down at the gym clothes I was wearing. I glanced at the sink where my salad bowl rested from lunch. I looked across the house to the full-length mirror I said I wanted so I could see my full outfit but really wanted so that I could have a 360-degree view of myself to ensure all was perfectly tucked and folded in to increase the perception of perfect thinness at all times. I felt a bit of guilt that that statement had come from my mouth. Here I was trying to convince my daughter that fat is not an identity while my whole world was wrapped up in the idea that I'm fat.

We're not fat. We just have fat.

We're not wounded or broken. We've got stories with texture to them.

I'm working on intentionally and authentically reframing my view of the words I use, including the *F* word (fat). We're reminded in Proverbs that life and death lie in the power of the tongue.[1] The words we speak and particularly the ones we use as identity framing devices matter—and they matter quite a lot.

BODY POSITIVITY

In the last decade or so, the body positive movement has really taken off. I have watched in awe and appreciation as other women have come forward, declaring that the body standards that have been imposed on us are limiting. As a woman of faith, I'm heartened because I believe body positivity equips us to free ourselves from the trap of self-criticism set for us and allows us to get one step closer to seeing ourselves as God intended us to be. Seeing other women embrace their bodies—and not just some glammed-up, Photoshopped version—has tremendously helped me to see my own in a much more positive light.

It's taken some time, though. Because what I wasn't ready to do when accepting my imperfectly imperfect body was to throw my own health goals and habits out the window. I didn't want to get rid of my scale, or stop going to the gym, or even stop sipping those green smoothies that I've come to enjoy. Eventually I realized I didn't have to.

Body positivity doesn't mean that you forgo any body goals or just "let yourself go" (whatever that means to you). The core idea behind body positivity is not that we have to forget all about doing the things that are good for our physical bodies. It's about shifting the perspective behind *why* and *how* we do these things. It's about removing the burden of compulsion—the sense that we have to meet these standards or we won't be valued—and replacing it with love and a drive to truly be our best and healthiest selves, no matter what we look like or what the scale says.

Loving your body *as is* and recognizing it as good means that when you throw your sneakers on and head out for a walk, you're not spending the whole time watching your smartwatch to see how many calories you're burning. You're walking because it feels good to get your blood flowing. Or because the weather is beautiful and you want to breathe in the fresh air. Or because exercise is just part of your daily life.

Loving your body will propel you to treat it with compassion and appreciation. It will help you prioritize self-care so you can be a better you for your family and friends. It will take the angst out of food and exercise choices so you can stop the self-defeating cycle of dieting and extreme workouts that you hate.

Loving your body will allow you to see food as something beyond just calories in or calories out. It will help you recognize that nourishment is a good thing that was designed to be enjoyable.

Body positivity is just that: seeing your body in a positive light. It is learning that your body is valuable, but it doesn't *determine* your value.

> Your body is valuable, but it doesn't *determine* your value.

Messages all around us are designed to get us to think that we are not enough. But what if we are? What if our healthiest self doesn't match the BMI chart at the doctor's office? Can we love

220

ourselves even then? What if we aren't dying in the gym, but we feel tired and need a week off? Can we love ourselves even when the tight muscle mass softens a bit? What if we'd rather be outside with our kids, playing in the yard instead of going running? Or if we grab fast food on the way home from a long day instead of trying to conjure something yummy out of those wilting zucchini in the fridge? What if, through it all, we chose self-love instead of self-hate?

WHAT I WOULD TELL THE OLD ME

It might seem strange that a girl with a massive weight-loss story chose to write a book about love. But I'd contend that no message is more important than this one. So much of why we engage in health and fitness routines goes back to something that is by definition the exact opposite of love: fear. Those of us who have dined with desperation often find that the company of fear feels similar. Fear may seem like a protective big brother—hovering over us, speaking words of wisdom into our ears to help us avoid pitfalls. But unlike an older sibling who has experience to share, fear has no other perspective than our own to guide its advice. What we hear speaking inside is nothing other than our deepest anxieties, brought to life under the guise of rational thought.

For many of us, fear is what drives us to eat a salad instead of fries—*I'm afraid of getting cardiovascular disease and dying young.* It's what motivates us to head to the gym even when we're positively exhausted—*I'm afraid I'll lose all my progress if I don't try hard enough.* In some ways, fear is a helpful motivator. After all, I want my ever-fearless son to be afraid of sticking a fork into the electrical socket or turning on the stove. That type of fear might hold him back from doing something dangerous. Fear isn't always bad; like all things in life, balance is key.

But many of us don't just have moments of fear—we live lives defined by fear. My most frequent fear is going back to what I used to be. I'm still the same Jennifer—my brain is the same, the same chambers of my heart are pushing out the exact same type of blood as they did many years ago. The nails I just painted are growing from the same stockpile as the nails I had when I was 336 pounds. The feet supporting my now smaller frame are the same feet that held me up at my heaviest. I'm still me. Only, I'm not. Not exactly.

What *if* I returned to square-one Jennifer? What if I returned to 336 pounds? Would I simply have to stop living because I hated myself so much? No! If I were returning to 336-pound me, my only request would be that I could take with me the incredible truths I now understand. How different would my trajectory have been had I understood back then that I was worthy? How easily could my habits have changed if I had approached them from a compassionate stance, rather than a desperate one? What joy could I have spread to the world around me, if only my eyes had not been staring down at my feet all the time?

I wish I could put my hands on my 336-pound shoulders and shake me. "Jennifer!" I would say fervently. "You don't have to believe the lies that are invading your heart! Look up!

Look at that girl in the mirror. Don't you see how beautiful you are? Who told you that you weren't? Push back against that self-defeating deception! Don't you know that losing the weight won't make you any more worthy than you are right now? You're already worthy! Don't you know that you could lose *all* the pounds and still you would not be more loved than you are right now? You're already loved! Don't you understand that you are capable of great things? That you have a beautiful life ahead of you? That you have gifts and abilities and encouragement and inspiration to share with the world around you? Wake up, Jennifer!"

I spent so many years inside my own head, unable to make an impact in the lives of others because I was so consumed with feelings of worthlessness. Now Jennifer has woken up. And she invites you to wake up too.

It's time to separate fact from feeling. We chase some elusive feeling of perfection that *none of us have ever felt,* pursuing that over contentment and peace and self-love. Want to know a little secret? None of us will ever have a perfect body. Those body standards that define "perfect" are chosen by others and are designed to keep us believing the lie that we are not enough—often to sell us products that promise to provide a remedy for our imperfections. At the end of the day, though, we are responsible for how we choose to buy into those standards. If you're holding on to unrealistic and ridiculous expectations about what your body should look like and it's making you live in a constant state of self-loathing, you first need to recognize that this is totally normal. Then you've got to realize that this isn't healthy—at least long-term. You get to choose to change that.

If fear is keeping us in this state, we've got to look to the antidote to solve the problem. And the antidote to fear is love.

I've noticed that it's perfectly normal to associate women and love in every single context *except* when it involves ourselves. Women are supposed to love their spouses, their kids, their pets, their domestic duties, and their jobs, but women are not often encouraged to love themselves. In fact, we often make it a normal rite of passage for young girls and women to engage in a constant state of self-criticism. We tell ourselves horrible, discouraging things—some of which I've highlighted throughout this book. But we can flip the script and learn to speak to ourselves in a way that reflects love instead of loathing.

Perhaps the Beatles had it right: Love is all we need. Or maybe the Love chapter in the Bible did: The greatest of these is love.[2] When we finally learn to *love* our bodies and ourselves as we currently are—not some futuristic or imaginative version of perfection—we find freedom. A life of self-loathing promises no real reward. But a life of self-love? That's an entirely different story.

BALANCED SELF-LOVE

We're not talking about self-infatuation or a conceited kind of love here. This is obviously not a book about putting ourselves at the top of our love-list and letting everything else fall by the wayside. This is about seeing ourselves as loving products of creation and allowing ourselves to walk in our purpose with appreciation for who we are. It's about accepting our bodies so that we're not consumed by them. It's about experiencing love for our true authentic selves so that we then can *extend* that love to others. And loving ourselves can help us along our health journey in some surprising ways.

With self-love we can sustain good habits.

I've previously shared some of my issues with crash dieting and exercise plans. Crash dieting is usually spurred by our despising our current state so much that we are willing to dive full-force into any quick-fix solution that promises something different from what we're feeling in the moment. Again, we're embracing *feelings*, not facts. And here's a fact for you—pursuing health through steady, ongoing effort and good habits will help you appreciate what you've accomplished far more than a temporary fix will. If you don't have to work for something, most of the time you won't appreciate it anyway.

Health is a lifelong habit and should be a forever pursuit. I'm not talking about a fixation with skinny. Though we put a lot of value on "skinny," keep in mind that you can be totally thin and totally still die prematurely from a heart attack, a stroke, stress, or any of the other things that try to bring about our pending mortality. This lifelong pursuit of health is about a constant pursuit of a better you, a more complete you, a healthier you—a you that loves *you*, no mat-ter what circumstances life throws your way. Isn't that ulti-mately the best good habit we could cultivate?

Imagine a world where you are steadily becoming healthier, happier, more fit, and more confident. Now imagine not hating yourself in the meantime. Think of seeing *healthy* and *fit* not as goals reflected in the numbers on the scale but in terms of feeling happier about the way your body—whatever size it is—occupies the spaces you find yourself in.

Having a positive view of self allows us to walk through our journeys to good health in a way that lasts. Why? Because although the numbers may change on the scale and the jeans we slip into might take a little more coaxing to get over our hips, if we are truly in love with our bodies the way they are, we naturally *desire* to take care of them. And you can't fake this. You can't *pretend* to love your body or *hope* to eventu-ally love your body. You can't set it as a goal for a year from now after you lose the weight; it's got to be something you pursue every day, wherever you are. One thing I've learned in my weight-loss journey is that your first goal should not be weight loss; your first goal should be self-love. That leads to the best results.

It's not as complicated as we make it out to be. We care for the things we love—our cars, our houses, our children—because we've invested in them. When is the last time you invested in yourself? The business community uses the term "ROI," which means "return on investment." If you invest in loving yourself, you *will* see a return on that investment when it comes to your health, wellness, and fitness.

With self-love, we develop confidence.

I've got family baggage, and I'll be the first to admit it. Coming from a broken family that also struggled economically, it was rough growing up. I'll never forget overhearing what a distant family member said about me when she thought I wasn't in earshot: "What does it for Jennifer? Is she ever happy?"

I was eleven and should have been happy. I wasn't. Because even though I was only eleven, my body and my psyche bore the psychological trauma of a forty-year-old. When I talk about being bullied, I'm not singing the ballad that seems to be thoughtlessly thrown out by some. My experiences weren't a "she said something mean to me" type of bullying; they were deep, dark, and painful, more than I can depict in these pages. I internalized a lot; I ate to cope; and I became silent to mask my inner turmoil.

That comment made me bitter for a while in adulthood. *What does it for me?* But when I reframed my thinking, I recognized that not only did I have the answer—I *am* the answer.

I do it for me.

I *do it* for me.

I do it *for me*.

When I began a journey of self-love, I spoke words of life to myself. I reminded myself that I am beautiful, that I have a rich history that has made me who I am, and that I am enough, as is. As I developed this deep commitment, I slowly started to gain confidence. That confidence was a paintbrush to me. I used it to paint over the hurt of my past—over the sneers of classmates on the playground, over the snide comments from relatives who hardly knew me (much less the real me), and over the self-doubt and insecurity that had literally etched itself onto my skin. I painted and painted, and although my masterpiece isn't complete, I'm proud of the work I've accomplished.

It amuses me now when people say, "Jennifer, you're so confident." Because for so long, *confident* was the antithesis of who I was. Honestly, even now I'm much better at putting on the guise of confidence than I am at actually *being* confident. But it was critical in my journey to understand that confidence, like the decision to love myself, is also a choice. I learned that you do not have to *feel* confident to *develop* confidence. In fact, there's little in life that you get before you put in the work. You don't make six figures right out of high school—you put in the work to build your career. And you don't just find yourself being confident if you're a woman in twenty-first-century America—you put in the work.

You *choose* to love yourself. You *choose* to love your body. You *choose* to slip into that little black dress, slide into those pointy-toed kitten heels, pucker those lips, and say, "Hey, world, whatcha got for me today?" And while you're *doing*, you're *practicing*. You're practicing boldness, even when you don't feel bold, and you're holding your head high, even though you might still see yourself "low." But here's what happens: The more you practice confidence, the more natural it feels. Eventually you stop looking in the mirror and saying, "*I believe* I'm enough," and you start looking in the mirror and saying, "I'm enough." As practice yields its fruit, those beliefs turn into reality. And before you know it, you've loved yourself into a new skill that sets you apart and will propel your future—confidence.

With self-love, we discover what our bodies are capable of doing. One thing I've learned throughout my health journey is that my body is capable of doing much more than I thought it could. As women, we're naturally trained to fold in upon ourselves. Think of the differences between a man and a woman on a train or a plane. Whereas a man will typically spread his legs and occupy as much space as he pleases, a woman is trained to believe that she should occupy as little space as possible. She folds her legs, tucks her purse under her knees, crosses her arms, and constricts her body as much as possible. We carry this physical response mechanism deep inside of us too. We're taught to be meek, mild, and quiet. This is especially true for those women who do not fit within the (toxic and often unattainable) cultural standards of beauty. We're taught that our bodies don't belong, so we conceal them (with baggy clothing), we constrict them (hello, Spanx!), and we try to camouflage them (black *is* slimming, you know).

Don't believe me? Ask any "fluffy" woman who's dared enter the gym. I remember the first few times I tried at my heaviest. Getting past the stares was hard enough (and there were enough stares to keep me away forever), but getting past my internal hatred was nearly impossible. Before I ever set foot on a treadmill or a StairMaster, I had psyched myself out. I needed to "get out of the way" of other people, I told myself. *Don't hog the machines; let the other people who regularly use them have them.* As if I didn't belong, and as if my pursuit of fitness was less legitimate because I didn't fit some standard. As if the gym rats could smell the brownies on my breath.

Though I didn't have much confidence at that point in my journey, I am so thankful I pushed those thoughts aside. I kept going. I stepped on the machine. I walked. Then I jogged . . . slowly. I jogged again, this time faster. Then I picked up a dumbbell (I dropped it, but hey, I picked it up). Then I added weights. Then I found myself peeking in the door to a group fitness class. Then I found myself in the back row. Then, front and center, five or six days a week.

And I'm so proud of the things I can now do with my body. I tuck-jump. I burpee. I high-knee-run/tuck-jump/jump-lunge until I want to puke—not because I feel like I have to but because I'm addicted to seeing how I can push my body to its limits. I do it because of the high I get by realizing that my body doesn't control me—I control my body.

This self-love-fueled journey isn't only about seeing what my body can do in the gym. I've also learned what my body can do in other spaces. Yes, my body with love handles, loose skin, and fat can wear a two-piece bathing suit to the beach.

Not everyone may appreciate it, but my body can do it and do it well. My body can carry my two babies (both giant lugs of things, like me and their dad) and tussle with them on the floor. My body can give a hug to a friend who's upset or lend a hand to someone in need. My body can do it all. I am amazed by her. I love her. I can't wait to see what else she does with her years on earth.

> My body can do it all. I am amazed by her. I love her. I can't wait to see what else she does with her years on earth.

With self-love, we give the world permission to love.

I don't mean to come across as rude. But, my friend—I do not need your permission to love myself. It's irrelevant to me. I'm thirty-something years old, and if my mom called me up today and said it was okay for me to skip my nap, I'd say "Um, okay. Thanks, Mom. That's awfully nice of you." But I certainly wouldn't let it dictate whether I did or did not nap.

I don't mean that you don't matter. You do matter, and you matter a whole lot. But one area where you don't matter is when it comes to *my* internal affairs. And nobody else matters when it comes to *your* internal affairs.

For a very long time, I waited around wishing and hoping that people would see me. Would understand me. Would validate me and tell me my worth. I waited and waited. Every now and then someone would try, but what I had to learn the hard way was that none of these outside influences would ever penetrate my heart until it was ready to hear the truth they were speaking.

Once I was ready, I made the choice to love myself. And now I won't sit around waiting for anyone to give me permission to see myself through a lens of love. When I choose to do that, I freely welcome love from others rather than inadvertently pushing them away.

People who refuse to see their own value are sometimes like porcupines. Have you ever tried to give a porcupine a hug? That's what it's like to be around someone with self-hatred. They may not even recognize it, but they wear their inner turmoil and loathing like a body suit as they interact with the world around them. And often, those people are not only incapable of loving themselves but are also incapable of loving others.

I remember a girl in my church youth group. She was a beautiful, freckled, strawberry blond with curls (hard to pull off in hot and humid South Florida!). If her beautiful smile didn't capture you, her vibrant energy would almost immediately. I watched from afar for a while before finally mustering up the courage to tell her that I thought she was incredibly beautiful.

Sweet gesture, right? But I was so caught off guard and immediately frustrated by her response: "Thank you. But I don't like when people tell me that. I just don't believe them, and I don't think it's true." Excuse me, what? You have the body I want, the smile I want, the personality I want, and the friendship army that I thought would fix all my problems. And you don't think it's enough? What is wrong with you?

The unfortunate reality is that it's hard to let people love us. And, as a consequence, it's hard to *feel loved*.

We need a fundamental shift in our perspective. I don't need your permission to love myself because—and hear me here with fierce gentleness—*You don't factor into my self-love at all*. You can't. Because if you do, that would mean it isn't *self-love*. It would depend on outside factors.

But just because I don't *need* you doesn't mean I don't *want* you.

We are sharpened by those around us. I am the product of a community of people who have had my back all along the way. They didn't make me who I am, but they supported me as I became who I needed to be. It isn't good for any of us to be alone; this is one of the core laws of humanity and the reason why intimacy, relationships, and friendship are so vital in life. Community is important because *connection* is so important. As humans, we have an innate desire to connect with others. As we share our stories, we expand others' thinking and have our own expanded. We show each other how our experiences alone cannot define the world, and we help give context to life's trials and its victories.

This is why self-love is so important. Imagine living in a *context* of self-love, in a thriving communal ecosystem where the guiding principle was to love yourself—to not only be okay with your flaws but to embrace them as part of the texture and fabric of life. Our self-love can inspire others to be who they are and to not feel limited by some imaginary, futuristic, "more perfect" version of themselves that may never be. We can make an intentional effort to build this ecosystem, to live by example, and to teach those around us how to love themselves and us.

We don't need to wait around any longer for permission. We can choose to love ourselves. And in doing so, I know we'll love others better too.

SELF-LOVE STARTING TODAY

You are not defined by your body, my friend. That means that all women—thin or stout, saggy or perky—are on the same playing field. What differentiates us? What brings texture to this tapestry of life?

I believe that loving ourselves allows us to lean into what makes us beautifully and uniquely amazing rather than squeezing ourselves into a society-designed box. No matter where you are on your health journey, know that no progress you make toward your goals can earn you more love than you already have.

So today, focus on loving your body as it is *right now*. Sense the history you've carried in this body—your romantic relationships, your children, your own childhood. Go grab that scale and stand on it proudly. Look at the number—love it and embrace it. Look at your naked body in the mirror. See those thighs as powerful. Appreciate that soft pouch on your tummy. Giggle a bit! Life doesn't have to be so serious.

And then laugh louder. Laugh without fear of your future and laugh at the idea that all of this that you see in the mirror could ever be defined by some newsstand magazine–fabricated standard of beauty.

Your body is good. You're beautiful. Now. Without ever changing a thing. You got it, girlfriend.

Now put your clothes back on and go out and show them what you're made of.

Flip the Script

Instead of telling yourself, "I hate my body so much," say this instead: **"Today I choose to love my body as it is."**

Reflect

What holds you back from loving yourself? What is the biggest obstacle you face? How could a healthy self-love change the way you react to those around you?

Action Step

Take a few minutes to jot down all the reasons you're thankful for your body.

Chapter 12

LENS OF LOVE

Early one morning, as I made my way down to the lobby of the hotel I'd been staying at while finalizing this book, I stepped onto the elevator just before a woman who was waiting behind me. I pressed the button that would lead both of us to the first floor of the building. Still waking my brain from a solid night of sleep, I waited silently. As the floor beneath us began to sink, I couldn't help but notice out of the corner of my eye what this woman was doing. During the entire fifteen seconds of our elevator ride, she evaluated her body in the reflective material that lined the walls around us, adjusting herself in response to what she saw. She straightened her posture a little. Brushed her hair out of her eye.

She took a full survey of herself, then put her head down, slumped her shoulders over, and waited until she heard the little ding that signaled we'd reached our desired floor. In those few seconds, she experienced the full emotional scale of what defines many women's entire lives—anxiety over a misalignment with assumed standards, panic to do anything as quickly as possible to meet those standards, and, finally, an overwhelming sigh as she realized that try as she might, she still didn't reach the standard.

I couldn't help but wonder what she was choosing to believe about herself as she examined her body. Was she wondering about her clothing choice that day? Whether or not she should have worn Spanx? Was she remembering some harsh words that had been etched into her heart and now coursed through her entire biological and psychological system? Was she wishing she could lose a few pounds? Did she feel inadequate? What was her inner dialogue as she stood there waiting, thinking no one noticed her eyes scanning every inch of her body?

Most of all I wondered—did she think it was just *her?* That she was the only one feeling like she didn't measure up?

I saw myself in her because I do the exact same thing. I use every mirror as an opportunity to critique myself. First, my eyes measure how much fat I have that day; I have pupillary precision to a fault and can tell without stepping on the scale if I'm up two pounds or down five. Once that's complete, I look at my hair to determine whether it's time for a trim or a new color. Am I thinning? Ugh, the one part of my body I *don't* want thinner! Then I look at my arms, where I'm definitely *not* thinning, and continue to bear witness to the pockets of fat that used to be there.

If I'm feeling good, I'll stand a little taller and flash a smile to myself. The chipped front right tooth doesn't bother me too badly most days, but the wrinkles around my eyes remind me that I'm not getting younger. Am I too old for this outfit? I pick apart every detail about myself until I have gone through the checklist that exists in my head. I'll call it a day when I've completed my due diligence and ensured that every space and place on this body that I call home knows I'm not happy with it.

And that's where I have to ask myself the big question that's been lingering in my mind as of late.

What would my life be like if this whole weight thing *had never* been a thing *for me?*

MY POST-BABY BODY

My weight has been a thorn in my side since as far back as I can remember. It's never *not* been a thing. Through every high and low, it's been a part of me. Take the high of pregnancy and birth and then the low of the postpartum period, for example.

When I was pregnant with my daughter, Kennedy, I watched my smaller-than-before body gradually get bigger and bigger. I panicked that I would end up right back where I started at 336 pounds years prior. I reminded myself often that I was growing a human, and it basically took superpowers to do such a thing. But those reminders couldn't erase the decades of weight struggle that told me I was destined to be fat forever.

As we reached and then passed my due date, Phil and I were finding it pretty hard to wait. When my water broke at 4:57 on that rainy Sunday morning, I felt anything but glamorous. I remember screaming "Oh my gosh, finally!" across the room at my husband, who had dragged our mattress out to the living room so I could find some version of comfortable in my eight-days-late pregnancy misery. We kicked the pizza boxes from the night before (yes, boxes *plural*— don't judge) out of the way, scooped up our packed bags, and headed to the hospital on our last day as just a couple. Many hours later—hours defined by epidurals, contractions, tears, stress, and weeping and gnashing of teeth—all my pain and pregnancy misery was worth it. There she was: sweet Kennedy at just under eight pounds. Beautiful big eyes and a head full of hair. (I *knew* it wasn't all that pizza that had given me the heartburn!) She was here, and she was perfect.

For the first couple of days after birthing Kennedy, I felt such a sense of relief. After carrying a literal human inside my body for all those months, it was an appreciated change of pace to send all those pregnancy symptoms fluttering out the window as I welcomed my sweet new bundle into the world.

When we finally got home and settled, all I wanted was to take a hot shower and put on some big, loose, comfortable clothes for my first night at home with our little bundle of joy. I climbed into the shower and every care evaporated away with the steam that filled the entire bathroom. But it wasn't long before the baby was crying and Phil poked his head into the bathroom, looking at me with question marks floating over his head. I told you, we were new at this whole baby thing.

I quickly climbed back out and grabbed the nearest towel to wrap around me. I dried off the best I could and tossed the towel aside so I could air-dry while searching for some clothes to throw on. As I reached down to grab one of Phil's T-shirts, I caught a glimpse of my reflection in the mirror. What was initially a blissful moment basking in the peace of a steamy shower quickly turned into heartbreak as the reality of my weight struggles returned to greet me. They'd given me a few days of relief while I was birthing a human into the world, but how dare I think they'd disappear completely. Cue the rush of defeating thoughts.

- *Before becoming pregnant you'd lost 100 pounds. Now look at you.*
- *You'll never get those pregnancy pounds off.*
- *No time like the present; better go on a diet. Make a meal plan for this week right away.*
- *Why is your tummy so loose and flabby like that?*
- *You're always going to struggle.*
- *You're never going to overcome this.*

Here I'd just done a superhuman thing, and all I could think about was how ugly my body was. Who the heck even cared?! Um, no one. Except me.

Self-love was not my initial reaction to my postpartum body, and I know I'm not alone in this. Women who have just given birth have done something incredible, yet often all we can think about is how ugly our bodies are and how soon we can get back to "normal." Why is it so hard to appreciate what our bodies have been through and what they've accomplished? They nourished a living being for nine months! They gave birth to a tiny human—no matter whether that birth went according to plan or met our expectations. Honestly, we should just relax and love our sweet babies instead of succumbing to the pressure to "bounce right back" to our pre-baby bodies.

I knew all that—and yet when my son was born a few years later, I went through the whole thing again. On top of all the normal concerns and challenges of pregnancy, I was also worrying about how much weight I would gain. Worrying about getting the weight off after he was born. Worrying about how many new stretch marks I would acquire or whether my skin would ever recover. Wondering what my new "normal" would be after the birth. Would I want yet another baby after this one? How would my body handle the constant drastic changes I was putting it through? I experienced such joy and excitement with this new life, but my weight was always in the background.

After all these years, it's as if my weight battle is ingrained in my DNA. It's been an obstacle, but through hard work and constant vigilance I've mounted that obstacle. If my weight was a mountain, then I feel that I've climbed Kilimanjaro. I've succeeded!

Yet every day I remind myself that there's infinitely more progress to be made. I never forget about my weight—and I'll never *not* think about it. No matter how healthy my body is, my self-esteem will always trail behind. Even if I reach the ridiculous standards that the BMI chart in my doctor's office says I should, my heart will still beat this way. I'm still me—and yet I'm not. I'm a different me than I was and a different me than I will be tomorrow.

My entire health journey has been a love story in the making. Maybe it didn't start off looking that way, but just like in every good novel, the tough times have led to a greater love—in my case, love for myself and for others. Though I've wasted years wishing I could escape the hard times, I now see that the hard times were only refining me for what would eventually produce one of the greatest joys in my life—learning to love myself, as is. Learning to believe that my body, no matter what weight I'm at, is good. And learning how to share that self-love and body positivity with the world around me. Starting with my own family.

> The hard times were only refining me for what would eventually produce one of the greatest joys in my life—learning to love myself, as is.

MORE IS CAUGHT THAN TAUGHT

After my kids were born, I learned quickly that moms have to deal with a lot. As if the endless cycle of dishes and laundry and sleepless nights isn't enough, we also serve as the

Directors of Communication for our families. No one is asked tougher or more questions than we mamas are. Case in point, the ever ubiquitous, "Why, Mommy?" If I had a dollar for every time I've heard that question over my ten years of motherhood, I could afford the babysitter I so desperately need for some time off from these children! Both of my kids are especially talented at their journalistic inquiry. I swear they'll both end up working for a news agency one day.

"Why do kids *need* to brush their baby teeth if they're just going to fall out anyway?" I don't know, Kennedy. Good question.

"Why *can't* I eat this mud patty I made?" Hmmm . . . good question, son. If it means I won't have to cook as much dinner tonight, go ahead and have at it.

"How should I sit so I don't look fat for the camera?"

Wait . . . what? My heart began beating harder in my chest when my daughter, just six years old, asked that question on a generic Saturday morning while I tried to snap a picture of her and her brother wrestling playfully on the floor. My phone and my stomach dropped together in perfect harmony.

"Why in the world would you ask that?" She shrugged it off and quickly bounced back into her giggly self. I knew full well, though, that it had begun. She was only six, and her worries should have stopped somewhere around the "Can I watch just a few more minutes of TV?" or "What am I going to get for Christmas?" mark. She'd hadn't even lived 2,200 days on earth but had somehow already begun her transition out of the magical land of carefree childhood and into the land of body anxiety that, at some point in their lives, comes to define the journey of every woman and girl.

This unhealthy self-view is prevalent in our society—and in ourselves, if we're honest. So if we're going to avoid passing it on to our kiddos and other young people around us, we're going to have to be intentional and think like educators.

And it's hard.

You don't realize how much you pull at your clothes, say mean things about yourself, or talk about calories until you have kids watching you. I can look my daughter in the eyes and wholeheartedly assure her that she is the most perfectly beautiful girl who ever walked the face of the planet—and believe it!—but if she constantly sees me taking a thousand selfies to get the skinniest angle possible, she's going to do what I do and not what I say.

We can't hide our struggles. Our kids and other children in our lives are looking to us as examples, even when they don't know it. They're going to adopt our patterns—good or not so good—because of the years and years that we spend together before they go off into the world to be grown-ups. We *shouldn't* hide our struggles. We'd be doing these kids a disservice if we didn't show them that in life they will have many troubles that come and go, but they will have the strength to overcome them all.

So instead of striving to completely erase a lifetime of struggles in a particular area, let's work one step at a time to chip away at our body issues in a healthy and sustainable way and show others how they can love themselves.

EDUCATING THE WORLD AROUND US

The world needs some "education." They need to know that it's perfectly fine for a curvy girl to rock a swimsuit. They need to know that not all fit people look the same. And they need to know that internal love and confidence are not a direct reflection of how we do or do not subscribe to some social standard of beauty or womanhood.

But this isn't only about educating some ambiguous crowd known as "the world." This is about educating "our world"—those we interact with on a regular basis. Maybe for you it's your coworkers, neighbors, circle of friends, or small group. My world is pretty small. So when I think about educating the world around me, I think about *my family*.

From the time I started *thinking* about having kids, I immediately wanted to spare them the turmoil that I had experienced. I was so focused on ensuring they would eat healthy foods and never struggle with their weight. But have you ever tried to feed kids healthy meals? Any honest parent will admit that it's not an easy feat. And it's not realistic. And it's not healthy.

Yes, feeding them healthy food is important. We want to get them the nutrients they need to grow strong. We want them to develop good habits and palates that accept more food than just chicken nuggets and mac and cheese. But it's not healthy to focus so much on your child's weight, living vicariously through them so they avoid the teenage turmoil you had.

Whether or not you have your own kids at home, you have children and adults who are influenced by the things you say and do. Let's be intentional about it. I'm working to ensure that my children understand that they don't have to fulfill anyone else's expectations of them. I'm working to ensure that my daughter understands what self-love is and how to practice it in a healthy way. I'm working to ensure that as I expunge my brain and identity of the limitations people have placed on me because of my weight and size, that I am not unintentionally filling Kennedy's brain with these discarded thoughts.

I do not want my kids to see me looking in the mirror and frowning at my rolls. For anyone who has kids and understands the harsh reality that you lose all sense of privacy and dignity, that means not looking in the mirror and frowning at those rolls. I don't want my kids to talk negatively about themselves or their bodies; that means I've got to stop talking negatively about mine. I don't want my kids to avoid certain places, spaces, or activities because they are worried they don't fit in them. So that means I have to be vulnerable and willing enough to intentionally insert myself in spaces that bring up old memories or uncomfortable feelings.

Let me say this: It's not our job to educate everyone we come into contact with. Women already carry heavy burdens and expectations that they will serve the world around them. I'm not about to add to that burden. My job is to educate my children. Yours might be to educate your own family or someone else in your circle. But even when it's not our job to educate others, one thing my journey of self-love has taught me is that when we love ourselves, we open up a lot more room in our hearts to love others.

LOVE WITHOUT LIMITS

Love in general is the key to moving forward in confidence. It's what allows us to work toward becoming the healthiest versions of ourselves, motivated not by desperation or self-condemnation but because we love ourselves and know our bodies are good. It's what fuels us in our journey to become healthy in every sense—not just in our bodies but also in our thoughts and attitudes.

My faith carried me through storms that were so dark they seemed like the end. My hope compelled me to put one foot in front of the other and to take steps toward becoming a better me. And though faith, hope, and love have carried me far, I'm reminded that the greatest of these is love.[1]

Love embraced me when I was at my worst. When I finally succumbed to the pervasive notion that I was unlovable, love came out of nowhere and showed me I was wrong. Love wrapped its arms around my 336-pound body, expecting no apologies or changes. Love didn't require payment or justification. And here's the thing about love—love would have been there if I had never lost a pound. Love was there all along. I just didn't see it because my eyes were stuck looking at a mirror of self-evaluation. I couldn't see love, but I'm so thankful that love saw me.[2]

There is too much life to be lived for me to get stuck in self-loathing. Too many invaluable moments to cherish with my family. Too many mornings to wake wrapped in the arms of my husband (or tangled in the feet of my toddler). Too many people around me who need encouragement as they navigate their own doubt-filled and seemingly hopeless health journeys.

So I lift my eyes from the nagging urge to critique myself, and I fix them on something other than just *me*. I reach into my handbag and pull out a pair of glasses that I should have been wearing all along. These are different because the lenses are filtered with love. When I wear them, I can relax my shoulders from the tense obligation that hounds me to see my flaws. When I wear them, I see people in a light of compassion. When I wear them, I don't fear that those around me are critiquing me. When I wear them, I can stand a little taller, smile a little truer, and love a little deeper.

Love reminds me to be patient. It doesn't hurry me along or demand perfection. It takes the steady road of developing roots that cannot be easily dug up. It focuses on today's part of the journey, never overwhelming me with what will be required tomorrow or in the years to come.

Love fills me with kindness—toward myself and toward others. It gently reminds me to talk nicely to and about myself. It sees me as perfectly imperfect and challenges me to see that as a good thing. Love shows me that I cannot

Love shows me that I cannot extend grace toward others if I do not first extend it toward myself.

extend grace toward others if I do not first extend it toward myself. It teaches me that kindness starts as a seed within my own heart, and then flourishes into the lives of everyone around me.

Love saves me from the slippery slope of comparing myself to others. It shows me the beauty in my own journey and keeps me from flaunting my victories in the faces of friends and foes. It trades pride for humility and a desire to serve in ways that add true value. Love prompts me to celebrate others and to honor their efforts. Love challenges me to take my eyes off myself and my own struggles, because it understands that change happens when we love others.

Love steadies my heart as I continue on my health journey, working to be the best version of me I can be. It calms the despair that rages in me when I fail. It doesn't tally my mistakes and then use them against me later. It reminds me to trust in the adventure of it all and to keep starting again. Love reminds me of the truth about who I am and where my value is derived from. It protects me from the desire to give up and causes me to persevere when I'm weak. Love gives me a glimpse of what's to come, and I do not lose heart.

Love is a gift that I am eternally thankful for. I see its value. I understand that my life would be nothing without it. And though it has taken a lifetime to wrap my brain around its infinite wonder, I cherish love so much that I cannot fathom living a day without it. I crave it. Unquenchably. And as such, I must extend it.

Love's impact transcends what can be seen with the human eye. It trickles out from an overflowing heart and softens the hearts of those it reaches.

I haven't always loved this journey that has consumed my life, but it's always been a journey of love.

Though many years have come and gone, I feel a fresh wind of anticipation for what is ahead. Because, while I once lay sobbing on my bed in a dark bedroom of desperation, my eyes now see the thing that will never fail me. The thing that will cause me to conquer any unexpected twists or turns. The thing that makes better anything it touches. The thing that I can choose to see when my feelings don't match the facts. The thing that has changed my entire life in a way I could never have imagined. The thing that will forever fuel my journey.

What would happen if you did the same? If you chose to dig deeper into that handbag, just like I did, and pulled out your own love lenses? I challenge you to do just that. To see yourself in in a new light, with a greater appreciation, compassion, and yes . . .

Love.

Without limits. Without conditions.

Love.

For you and from you.

Love.

No matter what.

Love.

Flip the Script

Instead of telling yourself, "I don't love what I see in the mirror," say this instead: **"I love myself without limits or conditions."**

Reflect

What would the world around you look like through lenses of love? How can you love yourself while still working toward goals in your health journey? Where do you find tension between those two ideas?

Action Step

Redefine your health goals while wearing your lenses of self-love. Write them down. Post them somewhere you'll see them often.

FRIEND,
YOU'RE IN A GOOD BODY

Hello, Friend,

As this book draws to a close, I wanted to take a second to speak directly to you—personally. I have attempted to make myself vulnerable in an effort to get you to realize one simple truth: You don't need to change anything about your body to become any more worthy or lovable than you are right here and right now. I'm a huge advocate for healthy, and I will always encourage you to pursue progress in the aspects of health that matter to you. Yet no matter where you are on your health journey, you are fully beautiful and loved. I'd do anything I could to make you realize this message. Climb the highest hill and swim the widest stretch of ocean—okay, that's dramatic, but in all seriousness, I believe so sincerely in the importance of this message that I would do anything at all to make you believe it at your core.

I've spent hundreds of hours pouring into the book you're holding in your hands. I've cried real tears recounting the experiences that crafted me as an adult who had to work really hard to overcome self-loathing about my body. Just under 70,000 words line the pages of this manuscript; and with each key stroke, I thought of you. While this book is filled with stories about me, it's also filled with affirmations and hope for *you.*

Reading a book won't magically overwrite the narrative in your head that tells you you'll never be enough. It won't erase the flashbacks of walks you've taken through muck and mire. As optimistic as I am, I know this will be a journey for you. You'll tiptoe forward with hopeful hesitancy. Some mornings you'll wake up, step onto the scale, glance in the mirror, and cry. Even though you're learning that your worth has absolutely nothing to do with any of the things glaring back at you, you'll forget sometimes. But once you get past the swell of emotion that relentlessly attempts to overtake you, you'll pick yourself up once more. And the real change comes every time you pick yourself back up and move forward with a renewed focus and renewed understanding that those moments don't define you.

While I wish I could swoop in and save you from ever again having a negative self-thought, I know for sure that this is a battle I am not able to fight for you. It's one that you must walk through. You will have to choose to believe that you are worth fighting for. And you *are*. You are worth the effort.

> You will have to choose to believe that you are worth fighting for. And you *are*. You are worth the effort.

Today and almost every day for the last five years I've been wearing the same necklace, a thin golden chain with a half-inch square as the pendant. I had it made specifically, just for me. On it, there are two words that have come to define the condition my body must achieve before it is deemed acceptable in my eyes. Much like a piece of furniture in a secondhand shop, I've got these two words hanging on me as a last-ditch effort to see the treasure in myself and to let that be enough.

These two words are tiny but powerful, and I want to gift them to you as you begin to blaze the trail of learning to love your body.

As is.

After you've tried and failed—to lose the weight, to fix your body, to fix your mindset—come back to this message. That you are perfectly fine and perfectly worthy, right here and right now where you are—as is.

My fingers grip this little reminder that rests just above the center of my chest, and I breathe a sigh of relief. *My body is good*—as is. Just as it is, my body woke up this morning. It pumped air in and out of my lungs. I'm able to move around. To pursue things. To love others.

No matter how many people have reduced me to my weight over the years, I now know that I am so much more than that. And so are you. You are free to pursue health in any way you wish—but you do not have to change one single thing about your body in order to start loving yourself. You are the one who gets to decide whether you will see your true worth or not. You get to craft your own standard of beauty. You don't have to turn your head and shy away from your body as it is today. And you certainly don't have to surrender to the lie that when people look at you, they see you as flawed.

What if they don't? Or if they do, what if you didn't care? What if the burden you've carried all this time was actually a wrong perception about yourself and about the people around you? What if the ones who spoke those harsh words were clawing for anything that would save them from the lies that were screaming in their own hearts and minds? What if the voices that reassured and affirmed you were actually the ones most genuinely truthful? Can you even imagine what life could be like *without* the grip of thinking your body needs to change before you can be happy?

This is my message—for *me* and for *you*. The world needs what we have to give, and that is reason enough to pull the blinders off of our eyes. Whatever is burning inside of you to share is needed. What you have to say matters. Your presence matters. Your voice matters. Your story matters. You are a gift! Push aside the lies you're buying into about your good body that are getting in the way of you walking out your purpose in life. Make a decision today to say "no more" and let yourself walk in the freedom of loving yourself enough to be enough, as is.

I hope you'll pursue all the things we've talked about in our time together. Move away from desperation and find a healthier motivation—your why. Take the risk to build relationships even if you're self-conscious about your body. Reject the idea that you need to be perfect to reach some unattainable standards of beauty. Define your health journey in your terms—set your own goals apart from the scale. Learn to love movement as a celebration for what your body can do. Nourish your body without falling into a defeating cycle. Embrace the fact that you will spend a lot of your life in the middle. Accept your scars and find a way to love them. View yourself through the lens of love.

As you close the pages of this final chapter, I hope you'll see it as a book still unwritten. I invite you to write the next chapter with me. Flip the script on your thoughts, ditching the self-condemning lines and instead speaking truth that reminds you who you are. With pen in hand and a renewed focus, let's write the next phase of our journeys, but this time in a healthy way. May they be journeys where we walk out our purpose free from the distractions, the lies, and the limiting views of ourselves and our bodies.

I look forward to reading your journey and watching you walk it out.

As is.

Together.

Love,

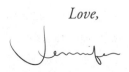

7-DAY MOVE YOUR BODY CHALLENGE

DAY 1: Ease into Things. Find three ways to move your body in a leisurely way today. In whatever way feels good to you, choose a time you'd normally be sedentary and replace it with easy movement of some sort. This could mean going for a walk, standing up for a few minutes after you've been sitting for a long time, taking a bike ride, heading outside with your kids or family, or doing some stretches on the floor while you watch TV.

DAY 2: Break a Sweat. Choose an activity that will leave your skin feeling dewy. This would be some form of movement that gets you slightly breathless. Once you feel the sweat starting to break, call it good for the day! This could be jogging, parking your car far away from the entrance of the grocery store, walking instead of driving, or taking the stairs instead of the elevator.

DAY 3: **Build Your Strength.** Let's get deep into the muscles on this one. Find an activity that may not leave you breathless but challenges you to work your muscles hard. This could mean taking a weight-lifting group fitness class, grabbing a couple of canned goods from your pantry and doing some bicep curls or rows, heading to your local gym, or simply moving some heavy furniture or boxes around.

DAY 4: **Use Your Body.** Your body is a fantastic tool for building fitness. Jot down five to seven exercises that require nothing but your own body weight. This might include squats, lunges, push-ups (knees or toes!), crunches, high-knee runs, burpees, skaters, planks, scissor kicks (lying on back), swimmers (lying on belly), crab walks, or calf raises. Do each exercise ten times in a row before moving to the next. Once you finish the list of exercises, repeat the list as many times as you want until you feel ready to stop.

DAY 5: **Stretch It Out.** Never underestimate the power of stretching your body. Find some time to center yourself and quiet your mind by doing some easy stretches. Remember, this doesn't have to look a certain way. Just get on the floor and try different movements that feel good to you.

DAY 6: **Build Intensity.** Let's really push ourselves today. Find an activity that challenges you physically and requires you to push past your comfort zone. This might mean joining a boot camp class, following a YouTube workout, or setting out for a vigorous walk or run. The goal today is to prove to yourself that you are capable!

DAY 7: **Breathe in the Good.** Today is all about moving in a way you truly enjoy. Find something that energizes you, brings you joy, and feels good in your body and mind. This might be taking an extended walk while you intentionally notice your surroundings or holding a good conversation with a friend. It might mean heading to a local attraction (like a park or beach) and committing to experiencing it fully. It may even mean trying that new fitness thing you've been eyeing. Take an inventory of what your body needs or wants today and lean into it!

30-DAY MIND/BODY CHALLENGE

One of my goals is to become the best and healthiest version of myself—and I want that for you, too. If you want to jump-start your health journey, try this simple 30-day challenge that touches on different aspects of mental and physical health. It will help you begin to clear out some of the negative body messages you've been holding on to, renew your thinking, and view your good body with love and appreciation.

1. Get outside
2. Completely unplug from social media
3. Send an encouraging text to someone
4. Order the book you've been eyeing
5. Turn on fun music and dance around
6. Go to bed a little earlier
7. Do a different workout
8. Declutter a closet or drawer
9. Start reading a new book
10. Take a bubble bath

11. Draw, sketch, or color
12. Indulge in something you enjoy
13. Go for a long drive with your favorite playlist
14. Watch the sunset
15. Take a leisurely walk
16. Give someone a compliment
17. Drink your water
18. Schedule a thirty-minute massage
19. Write a list of three body-positive affirmations
20. Unfollow people who spark negative feelings in you
21. Frame a photo
22. Go shopping by yourself
23. Power down your phone for the night
24. Do your nails
25. Break a sweat
26. Cook a yummy meal
27. Buy a fancy coffee or tea
28. List three things you're grateful for
29. Spend quality time with someone you love
30. Say three nice things to yourself in the mirror

SCRIPTURES FOR ENCOURAGEMENT AND INSPIRATION

Don't you realize that your body is the temple of
the Holy Spirit, who lives in you and was given to
you by God? You do not belong to yourself, for God
bought you with a high price. So you must honor
God with your body.

1 CORINTHIANS 6:19-20

Fix your thoughts on what is true, and honorable,
and right, and pure, and lovely, and admirable.
Think about things that are excellent and worthy
of praise.

PHILIPPIANS 4:8

We are God's masterpiece. He has created us anew
in Christ Jesus, so we can do the good things he
planned for us long ago.

EPHESIANS 2:10

Physical training is good, but training for godliness
is much better, promising benefits in this life and
in the life to come.

1 TIMOTHY 4:8

The Lord doesn't see things the way you see them.
People judge by outward appearance, but the Lord
looks at the heart.

1 SAMUEL 16:7

Thank you for making me so wonderfully complex!
Your workmanship is marvelous—how well I
know it.

PSALM 139:14

Don't copy the behavior and customs of this world,
but let God transform you into a new person by
changing the way you think.

ROMANS 12:2

ACKNOWLEDGMENTS

Many have asked what drove me through the long and intense process of writing this book. The answer is this: I couldn't *not* write it. Anytime I wanted to give up, a wind of encouragement would fill my sails, usually by way of someone who believed so fully in my message that they wouldn't let me quit. On November 7, 2017, I sat down to write, and the words poured onto the pages with ease. As I made my way forward, these incredible people landed perfectly in my path at exactly the right time, every single time.

Phil, you have been the exception to every presupposition I've had about what it's like to do life with someone. Through your words, your embrace, bouquets of flowers (or workout pants), boxes of tissues, and a thousand miles of walking in our neighborhood, you have been with me in every step of this process. You were the first person who spoke the words to my heart about writing this book. Before I could see it in myself, you saw the flame beginning to ignite. With gentle tenacity you fanned the flame until it was so bright that I couldn't put it out. This book wouldn't be half of what it is without you. Oh, how I love you.

Moses and Kennedy, it's hard to believe that at such young ages you had an impact on this project. I'm so thankful that our family is one in which words of encouragement overflow onto everything we set our hands to do. Thank you both for having no idea what it meant for me to write a whole entire book, but cheering me on as if I were truly changing the world. I love you both, more than words!

Kara, I knew you and I were meant to work together from the very first time we met, and I am eternally grateful that you were willing to take a chance on me. You have blown my mind time after time, but the most incredible thing to me is how well you have understood my heart. As such, you have helped me craft this message authentically and with zeal. Of the billions of people on this planet, I truly believe that you were the perfect person for the job. Thank you, thank you, thank you.

Karin, after our first meeting I was already thanking God for our partnership. Thank you for the countless read-throughs and for helping me steward this message. Thank you for leaning in when I changed directions and for soaking every edit in grace-filled affirmation. I have loved every minute of working with you, and I am so grateful to have had your expertise on this project!

To my incredible team at Tyndale House Publishers, thank you from the bottom of my heart! Working with you has felt a whole lot like becoming part of a loving, inspiring, encouraging family.

Christie McGuire, this book would not have become what it is without your presence in its foundational stages. For fixing commas, for believing in the message, and for undergirding a dream that has actually come true, thank you!

Mom, thank you for getting the most excited when I do even the tiniest thing. Dad, thank you for instilling a strong work ethic in me. Paul and Cindy, thank you for being a constant love and support. I'm thankful for the role that each of you plays in my life!

To Erika and Amelia, thank you for being the kind of friends who push me to go for it even when I'm not sure I have what it takes. For interrupting my writing times, for listening when I cried, for completing the perfect triad, thank you!

To Ray and Sharon McQueen, Jomo and Charmaine Cousins, Tony and Kaci Stewart, and Eric and Val Cobbins, thank you for watering our spiritual lives over the years.

To all those who were paving the way for body positivity long before I was ever blessed to learn this message myself, thank you! Thank you for changing the narrative, for being brave in your pursuit to challenge our thinking, and for living it in your everyday lives.

Most importantly, thank you, God. For quieting my heart when I wanted to run a thousand miles ahead. For surrounding me with people who would help me do the thing. For orchestrating what I could have never orchestrated myself in a million years. For doing far beyond what I could have hoped for, imagined, or dreamed of. For patiently walking me through a journey to see myself the way you do. For turning what was meant to crush me into something good.

ABOUT THE AUTHOR

JENNIFER TAYLOR WAGNER is challenging the way we think about health, wellness, and even weight loss. With her own massive journey to becoming her healthiest self, she is inspiring us to focus less on the size of our bodies and more on living free from the demands of diet culture. Whether it's leading groups of women, hosting online webinars, speaking in auditoriums, chatting at MOPS meetings, writing on her blog, or inspiring through social media, Jennifer is committed to helping us see that our current bodies are *good*, without changing one single thing.

Jennifer is a successful blogger at jennifertaylorwagner.com, where she delves into topics like health, wellness, fitness, body positivity, food freedom, motherhood, and the Enneagram (a personal passion). Jennifer is a certified fitness instructor through Les Mills. She is married to Phil, and together they have two children—Kennedy and Moses. They now reside in Williamsburg, Virginia.

NOTES

CHAPTER 1: BEYOND THE NUMBERS

1. See 1 Corinthians 6:19-20.
2. Emily Gerstell et al., "How COVID-19 Is Changing the World of Beauty," McKinsey and Company, accessed April 5, 2021, https://www.mckinsey .com/industries/consumer-packaged-goods/our-insights/how-covid-19-is -changing-the-world-of-beauty#
3. *Yare*, Bible Study Tools, accessed April 5, 2021, https://www.biblestudy tools.com/lexicons/hebrew/nas/yare.html.

CHAPTER 2: PERFECTLY IMPERFECT

1. Chris Jackson and Marie-Pierre Lemay, "Most Americans Experience Feeling Dissatisfied with How Their Body Looks from Time to Time, Including Nearly 2 in 5 Who Feel This Way Whenever They Look in the Mirror," Ipsos, February 13, 2018, https://www.ipsos.com/en-us /news-polls/most-americans-experience-feeling-dissatisfied-with-body -looks-from-time-to-time.
2. Mario Palmer, "5 Facts about Body Image," *Amplify*, 2014, http://amplify yourvoice.org/u/marioapalmer/2013/05/21/byob-be-your-own-beautiful.
3. Palmer, "5 Facts."
4. Deborah L. Rhode, *The Beauty Bias: The Injustice of Appearance in Life and Law* (New York: Oxford University Press, 2010), 41.
5. A. Gustafson-Larson and R. D. Terry, "Weight-Related Behaviors and Concerns of Fourth-Grade Children," *Journal of the American Dietetic Association* 92: 818–822, cited in "Perfect Illusions: Eating Disorders and the Family," PBS website, https://www.pbs.org/perfectillusions/eating disorders/preventing_facts.html.

6. J. I. Hudson et al., "The Prevalence and Correlates of Eating Disorders in the National Comorbidity Survey Replication," *Biological Psychiatry* 61, no. 3 (February 2007): 348–358.
7. F. E. Smink et al., "Epidemiology of Eating Disorders: Incidence, Prevalence and Mortality Rates," *Current Psychiatry Reports* 14, no. 4 (August 2012): 406–414.
8. Eating Disorders Coalition, "Facts about Eating Disorders: What the Research Shows," 2016, http://eatingdisorderscoalition.org.s208556 .gridserver.com/couch/uploads/file/fact-sheet_2016.pdf.
9. Eating disorders can happen to any of us. Women (and men) of all sizes walk through this struggle every single day. If you struggle with disordered eating or are worried that you might, you're not alone! Reach out to someone in your circle, a licensed practitioner, a support group, or The National Eating Disorders Association (which offers call, text, and chat support). You are not alone, and you are loved.
10. Chelsea Haynes, "True Cost of Beauty: Survey Reveals Where Americans Spend Most," August 3, 2017, Groupon Merchant, https://www.groupon .com/merchant/trends-insights/market-research/true-cost-beauty-americans -spend-most-survey.
11. "Real Girls, Real Pressure: A National Report on the State of Self-Esteem" (commissioned by the Dove Self-Esteem Fund, June 2008).
12. Thomas Curran and Andrew Hill, "Perfectionism Is Increasing Over Time," American Psychological Association *Psychological Bulletin* 145, no. 4 (2017): 410, https://www.apa.org/pubs/journals/releases/bul -bul0000138.pdf.
13. Ben Tinker, "The Modern Problem with Pursuing Perfection," CNN, January 9, 2018, https://www.cnn.com/2018/01/09/health/perfection -mental-health-study-intl/index.html.

CHAPTER 3: YOU GET TO TAKE UP SPACE

1. I believe we have an unnecessary fear of fat, seeing it in black-and-white terms. Either you *are* fat or you are *not*. When we do that, it's a real easy jump to label those identities as good or bad (and we know how that plays out). Let me be clear—all bodies have and hold fat. Thus, by default, we're all fat in some way; some of us more than others. So when I use this term, I'm not doing so in a denigrating way nor am I doing so in a way that refers to "old" (pre-weight-loss) me. It's easy to be critical of my use of this term and other before-and-after language, but please know that my intention is to facilitate an easy conversation.

CHAPTER 4: THE STARK NAKED TRUTH

1. S. N. Johnson and R. Engeln, "Gender Discrepancies in Perceptions of the Bodies of Female Fashion Models," *Sex Roles* 84 (2021): 299–311, https://link.springer.com/article/10.1007/s11199-020-01167-5.

CHAPTER 5: FREE AND UNFILTERED

1. Holly Furtick, "Shut Up and Shine," sermon given October 4, 2020, Elevation Church, https://elevationchurch.org/sermons/shut-up-and-shine/.

CHAPTER 7: MOVE YOUR GOOD BODY

1. Lysa TerKeurst, *Made to Crave* (Grand Rapids, MI: Zondervan, 2010), 69–76.

CHAPTER 8: YOU DESERVE TO EAT

1. "The $72 Billion Weight Loss and Diet Control Market in the United States, 2-19-2023," Business Wire, February 25, 2019, https://www.businesswire.com/news/home/20190225005455/en/The-72-Billion-Weight-Loss-Diet-Control-Market-in-the-United-States-2019-2023---Why-Meal-Replacements-are-Still-Booming-but-Not-OTC-Diet-Pills---ResearchAndMarkets.com.

CHAPTER 9: WELCOMING THE MIDDLE

1. Dictionary.com, s.v. "middle," https://www.dictionary.com/browse/middle?s=t.

CHAPTER 11: LOVE YOUR BODY (EVEN WHEN YOU DON'T)

1. See Proverbs 18:21.
2. See 1 Corinthians 13.

CHAPTER 12: LENS OF LOVE

1. See 1 Corinthians 13:13.
2. For some descriptions of the ultimate love God has for us, see John 3:16 or Romans 8:38-39. Nothing can separate us from his love! First Corinthians 13 also lists characteristics of love that I touch on below.

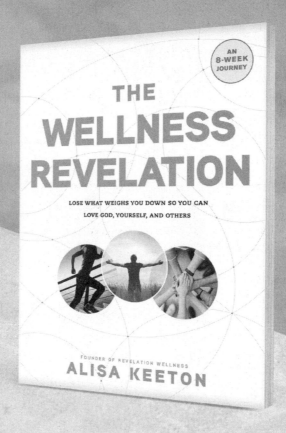